MEDICAL GENERALISM, NOW!

Medical Generalism, Now! is a unique and timely consideration of generalist medical practice. With a focus on the knowledge work of clinical practice and by taking a whole healthcare system view, the book responds to a recognised need to strengthen generalist practice within modern healthcare delivery in both primary and secondary care settings.

Through a series of creative provocations directed to consulting clinicians and their trainers/educators, service leaders and managers, and policy makers, readers are encouraged to challenge the orthodox view that generalism is an outdated 'jack of all trades' sub-set of clinical medicine delivering the 'simpler' aspects of medicine, with more complex issues requiring onward specialist referral. Case studies are used throughout to illustrate the challenges to be faced, accompanied by a description of the principles of generalist knowledge work needed to tackle the scenarios described and discussing the implications for practice and service redesign.

Essential reading for clinicians, managers and policy makers across all healthcare settings, the book concludes with a call to action, synthesising the learning from each chapter to define and describe delivery of the key changes needed.

Medical Generalism, Now!

Reclaiming the Knowledge Work of Modern Practice

Joanne Reeve

GP and Clinical Professor of Primary Care Research
Hull York Medical School, UK

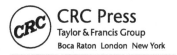

CRC Press
Taylor & Francis Group
Boca Raton London New York

CRC Press is an imprint of the
Taylor & Francis Group, an **informa** business

Designed cover image: Shutterstock

First edition published 2024
by CRC Press
6000 Broken Sound Parkway NW, Suite 300, Boca Raton, FL 33487-2742

and by CRC Press
4 Park Square, Milton Park, Abingdon, Oxon, OX14 4RN

CRC Press is an imprint of Taylor & Francis Group, LLC

ISBN: 978-1-032-28529-0 (hbk)
ISBN: 978-1-032-27290-0 (pbk)
ISBN: 978-1-003-29722-2 (ebk)

DOI: 10.1201/9781003297222

Typeset in Sabon
by KnowledgeWorks Global Ltd.

Contents

Preface

This is a book about the everyday work of medical generalist practice.

I am a practising clinician, with over 25 years' experience of generalist practice. Professional scholarship – including academic work – has been an integral part of my clinical practice throughout my career and has shaped the ideas and discussions in this book. But my goal was to write a very practical book. I have set out to challenge what I believe to be current outdated thinking about how we work, and so to spark within the reader a new vision for practice – today and in the future.

Perhaps it would help if I started by telling you a bit about why and how I came to write this book. Thirty years ago, I arrived at medical school with one pretty simple idea. If I could just understand things better, then I'd be better able to help.

I wasn't sure what I was going to help. My 17-year-old self at medical school interview probably hesitantly described some idea about helping people feel better. I wasn't too worried about what that meant in practice. I just assumed it would become clearer with time and experience. And to be fair, it has. But what has changed, completely, is my appreciation of what 'understanding' means.

Like many school leavers, I thought that if you wanted to understand something, you went and 'learned' about it. I am showing my age, but this meant reading the best textbooks, speaking with the best experts and remembering their pearls of wisdom. Understanding was about acquiring knowledge.

My early experiences at medical school started to open other doors. I began studying medicine before problem-based learning was established in the UK. Our first 18 months were spent often with primary scientists teaching us the basics of the applied sciences. I spent time in laboratories doing basic science experiments – which almost never went to plan. Most of the time, I thought this was because I was rubbish at doing the practical work (and that was certainly a factor). But I also started to recognise the limitations of the scientific method that underpinned all the 'facts' I was 'learning'.

After my second year of medicine, I took a year out to do an intercalated degree. I did it because I was thinking of leaving medicine – I wasn't convinced this profession was for me. I spent a whole year in a lab, working with a fabulous team on my own research project. Most of the experiments I did that year didn't work either – or certainly not in the way my supervisors and I intended – no matter how many times I repeated them with ever more careful attention to the details of the method. But what I later realised I had learnt that year was that understanding is created – yes, through careful attention to method, but with much more. And understanding is definitely more than knowing things. Although I didn't realise it at the time, this was to become the theme that would shape my entire career.

You will have gathered that I returned to medical training after my research year although with no intention of doing any more research. As I entered the clinical stages of my training, evidence-based medicine (EBM) was an emerging idea from a team in McMaster University led by David Sackett. Promising a new approach to enable and ensure 'the conscious, explicit and judicious use of current best evidence in making decisions about the care of an individual patient' was taking hold as a model for clinical teaching, and of best practice. My first thoughts were on the lines: Who could argue against that? And why was this something we weren't already doing?

I heard about a one-day conference at the Royal College of Physicians with David Sackett speaking on this new approach. It felt like I needed to be there, so I wrote to the conference organiser. I explained I was a student and couldn't afford their conference fee but would really like to attend – and they let me in.

My memory is of a powerful and eloquent vision of the future put forward by Sackett and his team. People in the hall voiced their anxieties about the risk of 'cookbook medicine'. Sackett ably diffused the immediate concerns. Yet for me, there was something missing – a problem, perhaps a flaw in the logic, that wasn't being discussed. I was troubled by what was being said – but halfway through my medical training, I had neither the experience nor the language to articulate what I was feeling.

Fast forward a few years, and I had joined the public health training scheme. Clinical medicine had frustrated me (again). It seemed that we fixed 'bits' but I hadn't experienced work to look at 'wholes' – the person beyond the broken part. My initial response had been to opt out of patient-facing practice and into public health medicine. Public health appealed to me because it paid so much attention to the context in which people become ill. But I soon hit problems again as I grappled with what felt like conflicting 'evidence' for practice. The science presented through EBM offered one view of 'best practice'. Yet, the science from patient-centred research offered a potentially different view. It felt like I was being asked to fit the square peg of patient experience into the round hole of EBM.

I was starting to learn the creative power of frustration! This time, I opted back into clinical medicine (general practice). I also signed up for a PhD to understand the knowledge work of whole person-centred care – a chance to critically explore how we can critically and safely go beyond the biomedical evidence prized in EBM to integrate the patient voice. My PhD gave me a language to start to articulate the discomfort I experienced as a student listening to Sackett. I learnt about concepts and tools that helped me start to build a response and an alternative. It sparked a career-long exploration of the ideas of generalism, and the generation of the work that is presented in this book.

This work helped me to recognise that we need a new approach to understanding, delivering and supporting whole person medicine. EBM has defined the knowledge work of clinical practice for decades: defining what data we use, and how we use it. EBM has contributed to improvement in professional practice and patient care. Yet, changing demographics, epidemiology and societal expectations of care mean that EBM is no longer sufficient for modern healthcare. Indeed, it may be contributing to iatrogenic harm through its contribution to structural iatrogenesis and epistemic injustice (concepts I shall return to in chapters 1 and 2). We need to look again at the knowledge work of medical professional practice – the way we find, create, use, generate and learn from data to do our everyday job. EBM changed the professional training, practice and system design for disease focused care. This book seeks to do the same for whole person medicine.

Change can be uncomfortable. In my 25 years of practice, I have repeatedly experienced how people's beliefs about medical generalism are integral to their professional identities. In this book, I will present a vision of generalist practice that may differ, at least in its emphases, from how you think about medical generalism. So, in Chapters 3, 4 and 5,

I will be sharing examples of my work which show how this different view of generalist practice is helping tackle some of the very real challenges we experience in our everyday work. I summarise what I have learned from this work to describe and explain the changes in professional training and organisation of practice that I call for in Chapter 6. Then in Chapter 7, I invite an international panel of colleagues to reflect on the ideas outlined in this book – the implications for their own contexts and indeed professional identities and any changes they would want to consider.

This book is unashamedly a call for change. I hope that this book can spark a movement, just as Sackett did all those years ago. EBM took off for two reasons. Firstly, because Sackett and his team were able to clearly describe a logical, structured approach to tackling the challenges of the day. But secondly, EBM also came at a time when there was policy and political will for change. Integrating EBM principles into policy offered scope to standardise and control medical practice in a way that hadn't been previously possible (as I will discuss in Chapter 5). The installation of EBM into healthcare policy shifted control over medical knowledge from the medical profession to external bodies under the control of government (currently the National Institute for Health and Care Excellence). The result has been a shift in the way we understand, train for, support and evaluate the knowledge work of clinical practice in today's healthcare. The unintended consequence has been a decline in whole-person-centred care, at a time when it is most needed to deal with the changing epidemiology facing our communities. The growing prevalence of chronic disease and multimorbidity, together with reduced capacity for whole person care all contributes to new and growing phenomena such as problematic polypharmacy, treatment burden and unmet need related to persistent physical symptoms. This book joins the growing international voices calling for a change in direction for our health services.

This book is also a blueprint for change. Whole person medicine, generalist practice, is not a new idea. Many people value the generalist approach. Many of you reading this book will already be using some of the skills described here in your everyday work. But 25 years of working in this field has shown me that for many people, medical generalism remains a hidden form of practice. Even experienced generalist practitioners struggle to describe what it is they do, often talking instead about using their 'gut instinct' backed by their 'relationship' with their patients. Neither idea is enough to support new practitioners coming into the field to confidently develop their own skills and practice; or to enable policy makers to design new models of healthcare delivery.

Therefore, this book sets out to make the work of generalist medical practice visible, just as Sackett did for specialist medicine. In the chapters that follow, I will describe a clear vision of the wisdom of whole person care – the distinct knowledge work of medical generalist practice. I will describe the specific changes in professional training, practice design and healthcare policy needed to support and sustain delivery of whole person healthcare. In this book, I therefore provide a framework by which we can deliver Medical Generalism, Now!

Joanne Reeve

Author

Joanne Reeve is an inner-city GP committed to clinical scholarship and excellence in academic primary care driving person-centred redesign of primary medical care services.

As Professor of Primary Care Research, she leads a body of work on innovative scholarship driving excellence in primary care. She established the Academy of Primary Care at Hull York Medical School, where she supports a range of research on person-centred care in the context of problematic polypharmacy, sleep management in dementia care and homeless healthcare. She works with a range of partners to establish a series of innovative projects including the WiseGP programme (SAPC and RCGP), the CATALYST programme for new to practice GPs (NHSE and HCV Primary Care Partnership) and the WISDOM project supporting clinician scholarship (HEE Yorkshire).

She has worked for 20 years as a salaried GP within inner-city practices in Liverpool and Hull, including leading innovative service development work addressing care for people living with multimorbidity and problematic polypharmacy.

She regularly teaches primary care clinicians and academics at all career stages and is privileged to be a mentor to future primary care leaders who continue to inspire her everyday work.

Additional contributors

Professor Jane Gunn
Dean
University of Melbourne Medical
  School
Australia

Dr Stefan Hjorleifsson
GP
Norway

Dr Koki Kato
Director
Madoka Family Clinic
Japan

Professor Kurt Stange
Case Western Reserve University
USA

Professor Chris van Weel
Radboud University
The Netherlands

CHAPTER 1

Principles of whole person medicine

Medical generalism is the expertise and practice of whole person medicine (Howe 2012). It stands in contrast to the expertise of a specialist medicine focus on condition or organ-system specific medical care. In a wide ranging, and sometimes confusing, literature on medical generalism, this distinction is perhaps the one common thread.

Despite this clear distinction between these two forms of clinical practice, it is interesting that the *roles* or *work* of medical generalism are often still defined with reference to specialist medicine. A generalist physician has been described as a 'jack of all trades' (Griffiths 2016). The generalist is seen as someone who knows a little bit about a lot (of medical specialties), and so can deliver many 'basic' aspects of care. The generalist general practitioner (GP), for example, is commonly seen as a readily accessible clinician able to coordinate multiple elements of (specialist) healthcare in the patient's own community context. The generalist role becomes defined as *managing* the 'easier' bits of specialist medicine and *referring* on the more complex elements to specialists. The work of the generalist is seen as care coordination, navigating patients through healthcare.

All of these roles are important components in an effective integrated healthcare system. But as we will explore in this book, these accounts are a misunderstanding and misrepresentation of the scope of work of expert medical generalist practice in a modern healthcare system dealing with the growing challenge of complex healthcare needs (Box 1.1). Drawing on 20 years of research and scholarship, this book will redefine the work of medical generalism for today's healthcare (Box 1.1).

DOI: 10.1201/9781003297222-1

BOX 1.1 WHAT'S IN A NAME: GENERALISM, GENERAL PRACTITIONER AND GENERAL PRACTICE

If we want generalist practice to be clearer, we need to start by clarifying some of the confusing terminology. These three terms – generalism, general practitioner and general practice – all contain the word 'general'. Perhaps that is why people often use the words interchangeably, talking about general practice when they actually mean generalist practice, for example. Each term refers to something different and distinct.

In the UK, general practitioners (GPs) are the largest group of practising medical generalists, but GPs also deliver disease-specific (specialist) healthcare. General practice refers to a community healthcare setting providing primary medical care – a 'general range' (rather than a specific focus) of healthcare services that includes specialist and generalist care.

I have often thought that it would be helpful to find a different word instead of *general*ist. But since it is still a commonly used term in Western healthcare, I start instead by clarifying the definitions of each of these terms as I will use them in this book.

General practitioners are clinicians trained in the medical speciality which focuses on primary care medicine. The terms *general practice* and *family medicine* are defined by the World Organisation of Family Doctors (WONCA) and, in the UK, by the Royal College of General Practitioners (RCGP). In this book, I will refer to general practitioners as GPs.

General practice is the community model of primary healthcare delivery in the UK. If I talk about general practice in this book, I am referring to the organisational unit. When talking about professional practice, I will refer to GPs.

GPs are clinicians with expertise in the distinct knowledge work of whole person medicine. GPs use both specialist and generalist skills depending on the problem presented to them. The GP meeting a patient overwhelmed by the number of different medicines they take for multiple long-term conditions foregrounds their generalist skills to reassess and re-prescribe according to a tailored assessment of need (see TAILOR in Chapter 5). A GP meeting a patient with crushing chest pain who is sweating switches on their specialist skills to assess the need for urgent cardiology care. The expertise of the GP is the ability to *oscillate* between these two forms of clinical practice (Hjorleifsson, personal communication).

In this first chapter, I want to set the scene for the detailed discussions that follow by outlining five principles for understanding whole person, generalist medicine:

1. The *purpose* for generalist, whole person medicine – creating a whole person understanding of illness.
2. The *focus* for whole person medicine – understanding the self who we care for.
3. The *goal* of whole person medicine – enhancing health as a resource people need for daily living.
4. The *work* of whole person medicine – the wisdom of understanding in context.
5. The *context* in which generalist medicine happens – delivering a complex intervention in a healthcare setting designed to support this work.

1.1 THE PURPOSE FOR MEDICAL GENERALISM: CREATING WHOLE PERSON UNDERSTANDING

I opened this chapter by stating that medical generalism is the expertise and practice of whole person medicine, but I also recognised that there is much confusion attached to discussions of generalism. So let's start by clearing the pathway to our exploration of generalist knowledge work by clarifying what medical generalism *isn't*.

I have been studying generalist medicine for over 20 years. I have heard many accounts of what the generalist is and does. I want to start by challenging three common stories offered about generalist practice. All relate to the way that generalist practice works, what it does. But each has lost touch with the defining purpose of medical generalism.

Not 'soft' skills, but the skills to deliver tailored care

Medical generalists look after the whole person, and so it is perhaps unsurprising that people often conflate generalist practice with the idea of person-centred care. But person-centred care is neither distinct to generalist practice nor sufficient for effective generalist practice. Let me explain why.

Harden (2017) recognises the person-centred approach to mean putting people, families and communities at the core of the design and delivery of healthcare. As she discusses, there are many elements to the delivery of person-centred care. In UK general practice over recent years, emphasis has often focused on the importance of interpersonal skills including empathic practice, consultation skills and relationship-based care – sometimes described as the 'soft skills' of practice. But specialist clinicians would, rightly, reject an assertion that person-centred care is the exclusive domain of generalist medicine. A cardiologist may focus on clinical decisions about the management of an individual's heart problem, but they will be engaged in conversations with a whole person about their goals, preferences and concerns. The clinical skills of communication, empathy and listening are not exclusive to generalist practice, and so do not define the expertise of the medical generalist. Generalist medicine and person-centred care are not synonymous.

Yet, these patient-centred skills matter – my own research and clinical experience confirm the therapeutic benefit of relationship-based care. But a patient in one of my previous research studies shows us why relationships and soft skills are not enough (Reeve et al. 2012).

Helen was a young woman in her fifties dying from breast cancer. Before her diagnosis, Helen was a busy wife, mum, working woman. Terminal cancer had turned her life upside down. Helen spoke movingly about her relationships with her clinical team. She described the empathic care she received from the range of health professionals involved in her care. The staff laughed with her, cried with her and offered her comfort. They were able to signpost her to help for the range of problems she faced as a result of her illness – the impact on her finances, her mobility and her everyday activities. Helen received great *personal* care.

But Helen was also very critical that she didn't receive *personalised* healthcare. The problems related to medical decisions about her treatment. Here, Helen had a very different story to tell. The same staff who had offered great personal care were also responsible for her medical care. Helen had decided that she didn't want to have any more active medical treatment, preferring to spend the time she had left with her family and friends – doing her everyday things. But she reported that staff repeatedly offered 'evidence-based' justifications for clinical decisions; they repeatedly asked her to consent to further treatment (palliative chemotherapy). Helen described that her clinical team seemed unable, or unwilling, to tailor care despite being so familiar with her personal circumstances. Helen described that in these clinical conversations, she felt like she was 'stuck on a conveyor belt'. All of the personal care was forgotten, lost. The impact was that healthcare conversations became a drain on her health for daily living and were not supportive.

Helen highlighted that person-centred (so-called 'soft') skills are important but insufficient for generalist, whole person, care. Instead, a generalist clinician must be able to *tailor* care (including the use of 'evidence') to the context of an individual. We will look in more detail at what this involves in Chapter 2.

No jack of all trades, but expert knowledge worker

When I started researching generalist care, I asked a group of GPs, 'How would you describe a generalist?' They almost all told me that a generalist is someone who knows a little about a lot of things. This allows them to deliver first-line care for the range of problems that patients present to them. They described themselves as a 'jack of all trades'.

This label has shaped perceptions of the generalist role, especially GPs, for some time. There is a common misconception that GPs work simply to filter and sort patients, dealing with the easier problems, and passing on the more difficult elements to specialist clinicians. The perceived skills needed to do this 'sifting and sorting role' focus on the tasks done (multitasking); the knowledge needed (a little bit about a lot); the interpersonal skills (empathy, communication, relationship-based care); and the values of the practitioner (empathy, advocacy, ethics). All of which has shaped the vocational training of so-called generalist GPs. Now, as GP numbers in the UK have diminished, the service has started to train up other professionals, including Advanced Clinical Practitioners, Advanced Nurse Practitioners and Physician Associates, in these same tasks.

But the reality of the work of whole person, tailored healthcare is much more complex. As patients live and present with ever more complex healthcare needs, staff trained for a jack of all trades role find themselves unsupported to provide the care needed by individuals. Consider, for example, a frail elderly person living with multiple long-term conditions. The jack of all trades generalist can try and coordinate the delivery of multiple disease-focused guidelines of care. Digital technology may aim to help them work more efficiently. But as I will discuss shortly, these approaches are leaving patients overburdened by healthcare, and staff burnt out in trying to deal with the disconnect between the job described by healthcare systems and the need described by their patients. Yet, if provided with the resources and support to use their distinct expertise, the medical generalist can do so much more. The expert generalist physician is able to create, deliver, review and revise a tailored management of healthcare that optimises the health of this frail elderly person so that they can maintain their daily living. This is the distinct knowledge work of advanced medical generalist practice, and it is the work I will champion through this book.

Not better integration but new design

The primary purpose of generalist medicine is to create a whole person understanding of illness so as to inform, shape and evaluate the healthcare that follows. It means that whole person medicine is much more than the efficient integration of specialist medicine (Lewis 2013). We need to rethink our approach to healthcare delivery.

My research has highlighted a number of contextual barriers to delivery of whole person, generalist healthcare. These studies have consistently highlighted four barriers: a failure to value, prioritise, enable and sustain the complex work involved in delivering tailored healthcare. As we hear repeated calls from health service leaders for changes in the culture of modern healthcare, we need to redesign our healthcare systems to address those barriers. This book outlines how we can.

1.2 THE FOCUS FOR WHOLE PERSON CARE: THE CREATIVE SELF

It is common to hear people talking about 'person-centred' care in many settings, but what actually do we mean by person-centred? I said there were multiple, often confusing, accounts of generalism – and the same is true of person-centred care.

In 2019, Professor Chris Dowrick led the publication of a new book on person-centred primary care. He argued the need to recover a 'sense of self' for both patients and professionals if we are to undertake genuinely person-centred care in everyday practice. The book looks at why concepts of the self matter not only to philosophers and academics, but to managing the practical challenges facing clinicians every day. These include mismanagement in clinical practice, dealing with technology in the consultation and addressing the epistemic disadvantage (experience of not being heard) faced by patients such as Helen.

My contribution to that book was a chapter on the role of primary care, generalist practice, called 'Unlocking the Creative Capacity of the Self' (Reeve 2019). This work was developed from Havi Carel's writing. Carel is a professor of philosophy living with a life-limiting long-term illness. In her writing, she invites us to recognise what she calls the creative capacity of every individual. Her work describes the innate capacity of every one of us to respond to the ups and downs of daily life, including the adversity of illness (Carel 2008). She invites us to consider the resources available to a person to do that work. For me, her writing sparked a recognition that as a healthcare practitioner, my job is to ensure that the care I offer enhances, perhaps even optimises, that capacity – but certainly doesn't undermine it.

Carel's writing challenges us to think differently, and more broadly, about what we – as healthcare professionals – are trying to do. The generalist clinician, seeking to deliver whole person care, needs to think not only about the disease(s) that an individual has but also the resources that they have for daily living with those diseases (including those that could be enhanced). Carel reminds us that medicine is only one (often small) part of healing, improving health. Carel reminds us that we should start our conversations, our consultations, with a curiosity about this person *in the context of their daily life*. We need to be curious not just about the illness, but also the resources and context that shape their experience of illness and its management.

Just as Helen described, a person who is ill is also a person living their daily lives. They are working to keep a roof over their head and food on the table, looking after family and friends and managing the work they do for an employer and for society. This so-called work of daily living goes further than those practical everyday tasks. Maslow described the many additional layers of work that people do every day – for example, in building and maintaining their self-esteem, their confidence and their sense of place and identity (Maslow 1943) (Figure 1.1). A person who is dealing with illness is also dealing with all of the context and work of daily life. Illness happens in context – and that context shapes not only the experience of illness but also the resources that someone has and needs to deal with illness.

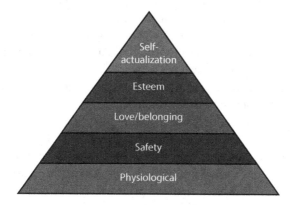

Figure 1.1   Maslow's hierarchy of needs.

There is a rich body of research describing the work people do to manage their daily lives whilst living with chronic illness. Clinicians reading this book will likely have been introduced to some of this work when you were an undergraduate in courses on health and society, social medicine and the behavioural sciences. These courses can introduce us to the 'whole person' experience of illness, although often with limited discussion of how those perspectives can be integrated into daily medical practice and decision-making. I will return to this point when I consider Iona Heath's work in Chapter 3.

One of the most influential areas of that work was started by a sociologist called Michael Bury. His research looked at how a new diagnosis of a chronic illness, in this case rheumatoid arthritis, impacted a person's story of their daily life – their biography. Bury (1982) described the disruption to everyday living caused by the effects of the illness, the treatments – medication and engagement with healthcare. He also recognised the impact of the diagnosis on an individual's identity and sense of self. Bury described the work that people do to adjust to now being 'ill', no longer healthy and possibly disabled with a new sense of their personal identity.

Other research followed looking at experiences in other communities and for other conditions. Some of these authors challenged Bury's account of the impact of illness (for example, Faircloth et al. 2004; Williams G 1984, Williams S 2000). They noted that a diagnosis of chronic illness wasn't necessarily disruptive to daily living. These studies described how some people can adapt successfully to the new element in their daily life that comes with an illness diagnosis. Faircloth and colleagues described this ability to restore and maintain their daily life as maintaining biographical flow. Later studies even described how illness can even bring positive change to daily living (Williams 1984). I saw one example of this in my research for my PhD (Reeve 2006). I was looking at people's experience of distress when living with a terminal diagnosis of cancer. One participant in my study was a young woman dying from ovarian cancer. Whilst she was fully aware that her cancer diagnosis was terminal, she spoke movingly about how being 'terminally ill' had transformed her from being an overworked undervalued housewife to someone who 'mattered'. A devastating (and highly disruptive) new diagnosis had also bought additional help in her work of daily living.

Understanding how and why illness impacts differently on individuals' daily living has significant implications for making healthcare decisions. The aspects of care that we prioritise, along with the elements of care that we put to one side, will be shaped by these personal lived experiences. These experiences shape the 'ideas, concerns and expectations' that consultation models such as the Calgary-Cambridge model asks us to explore with our patients. And indeed, we can simply ask people directly, What are you most worried about? Or, What would you like me to do today?

Personally, I have rarely found these to be very helpful questions in a clinical consultation. Asked directly, they often elicit a response along the lines of 'I want to know what's wrong with me' or 'You're the doctor ...'. Neither takes us much further forward in our exploration of an illness problem. But if I have first explored the everyday work that my patient is juggling, whilst also managing their health concerns, ideas about concerns and expectations become part of a discussion – the exploration – rather than a direct question. 'There's a lot going on there ... how are you managing to juggle all of this, deal with your hip problem along with everything else ...'

In person-centred primary care, I bring together Carel's work on the creative self, this body of research on the work of being ill, and my own clinical experience of working with people living with chronic illness to develop and describe an account of the creative capacity of the individual self. In my account of the Creative Self, I recognise five elements that influence our ability to deal with potential disruption to daily living created by adversity including illness. These are the Creative Self, the energy to Power the work of everyday life, the factors which offer Stability and which create Imbalance, all taking place within the context of a more or less turbulent Flow of Daily Life (see Box 1.2 and Figure 1.2). The chapter offers a series of case studies to explore how as a clinician, we can make use of these elements to shape our consultations with patients.

In daily practice, these elements offer me a series of pointers to explore in a conversation with the person who has come to see me about their illness. How steady, or indeed turbulent, is their everyday life just at the moment? What are the factors that act as 'anchors' or 'ballast' in this potentially choppy ride – perhaps the support of family or friends, the aspirations and goals that provide motivation even in the dark times or the beliefs and values that provide comfort? Indeed, when my conversation with a patient reveals that they recognise few or none of these, this will be ringing a warning bell in my head. I may go on to explore what factors are unsettling things at the moment – making it harder. Often these are losses – loss of family and friends, work, home and safety. I explore where my patient's energy levels are at – 'You sound exhausted' often opens up a frank discussion about how much 'power' is left at the moment. And through all of this, I am asking myself – and ultimately

BOX 1.2 CREATIVE CAPACITY

The *Creative Self* refers to the innate capacity of every human being to respond and adapt to a stimulus. It is the intellectual, emotional, physical and spiritual essence of ourselves that enables us to make sense of, and enact, daily life. Faced with illness, the goal for healthcare is therefore to enable the patient and clinician together to optimise the capacity of each creative self.

Each creative self needs resources to *Power the work of everyday life.* As described by Maslow, these resources are varied – whether the basics of shelter, food, warmth and the complex social activities of being with family, friends or in work. All can be both drained and restocked by the activities we do – including the health and health-care work. Resources can be enhanced through partnerships – including partner-ships with healthcare professionals. This doesn't mean that healthcare professionals taking on extra roles and responsibilities; but it may involve professionals in reducing the healthcare work 'required' from an individual whose resources are depleted.

The *Flow of Daily Life* recognises that illness work is just one element in the broader schedule of daily work we each manage. The tasks of living with illness, and of managing daily healthcare routines, all occur in the context of the flow of daily life. For some, this may be relatively calm; for others, and at other times, this may be turbulent. Any healthcare work we ask of an individual needs to recognise, and fit with, the broader flow of daily living.

Our daily task to navigate through the flow of daily life will be made easier or harder by the *(Im)balance of resources and demands* on an individual and their creative self. In 'Unlocking the Creative Capacity of the Self', I introduce John and George. John lives with type 2 diabetes mellitus and some significant complica-tions arising from that. But he also describes strong social networks, together with a strong personal understanding of his priorities and values, all of which help him to juggle the many healthcare-related demands on him. George has fewer biomedical complications from his diabetes but also fewer supportive resources to call on. George was at greater risk of being overwhelmed by the burden of his illness than John, even though his biomedical risks were less.

Finally, the creative self recognises that the things which matter to us as indi-viduals provide important *Anchors or Ballast* in managing the turbulence of daily life. Often these reflect our sense of identity, our values. A strong faith may be an important anchor; as may a strong sense of my role as a wife, friend and member of a group. Anything that disrupts those anchors may undermine an individual's creative capacity to continue to navigate the choppy waters.

More discussion on these can be found in Reeve (2019).

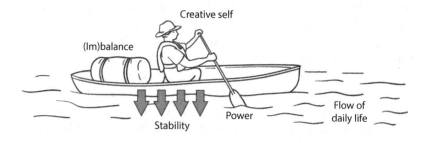

Figure 1.2   Imagining the Creative Self.

my patient – does this person recognise (feel) how much they are already doing in managing this illness problem.

When I discuss this concept with fellow clinicians, they have often questioned whether it is appropriate for clinicians to open up these wider conversations. They ask if there is a risk that by exploring these wider social and societal issues, that we may unintentionally be taking on responsibility for issues that are beyond the remit of medicine and healthcare; inappropriately extending the medical gaze further. I usually respond by suggesting that instead, this concept of the creative self helps me to be clearer about boundaries and what is not my role. By understanding the context and capacity of the creative self that is my patient, I am better able to understand if and when medicine may have something to offer *or not* for the problems they are presenting. These conversations help in recognising when medicalisation of illness problems (including, for example, investigation and referral) may not be appropriate – unlikely to benefit the individual and being more likely to burden or harm.

I find the concept of a creative self a useful way to highlight an understanding of the purpose of health as being to support everyday living – a means to an end, and not an end in itself. So let's look at that idea a little more.

1.3   THE GOAL OF HEALTHCARE: ENHANCING HEALTH FOR DAILY LIVING

The purpose of generalist healthcare is to understand the health and healthcare needs of an individual with creative capacity, enabling them to manage illness related disruption to daily living. This frames the goal of generalist healthcare – to enhance health for daily living.

The World Health Organization (WHO) has long advocated for an understanding of health in the context of daily living. WHO's asset model of health described that 'health is a resource for everyday life. Not the object of living. It is a positive concept emphasising social and personal resources as well as physical capabilities' (WHO 1986). Williamson and Carr (2009) developed this idea further in recognising health as a societal resource – a form of social capital that enable people to participate in society. When people have good health, they can participate in and give to society. Both the individual and the collective community benefit from investment in health capital. The authors intend to recognise health as a form of capital in order to encourage investment in a societal resource to be valued and nurtured for the public good. Indeed, the Public Health Agency of Canada describes health as 'a positive concept that emphasises social and personal resources, as well as physical capabilities'. So how do these discussions help us understand the goals of healthcare, and especially generalist (whole person) medical care?

Firstly, these definitions flag up that health is dependent on much more than biomedical factors. You will probably be already familiar with the public health model describing the social determinants of health (see Figure 1.3). I have already discussed Carel's work highlighting the (important but) limited contribution of healthcare to health and wellbeing. Dahlgren and Whitehead's (1991) model reinforces that understanding. Both perspectives highlight the limited role of medicine

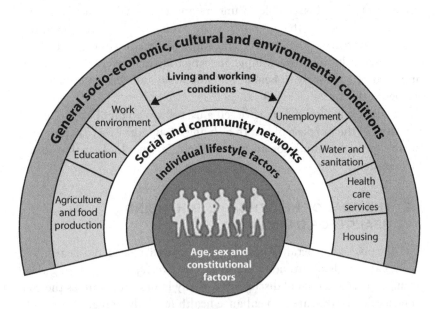

Figure 1.3   Dahlgren and Whitehead's social determinants of health.

in shaping the health of individuals and populations. Any medical decision has to be made in the context of this wider understanding of health.

The model describes the range of social, economic and personal factors which influence the health of an individual. Our overall health and wellbeing are shaped by a wide range of factors. Personal attributes and medical healthcare are both factors which may be considered in a healthcare setting. But the model also recognises the importance and contribution of many others including living and working conditions, social and community networks and general socioeconomic, cultural and environmental factors. All of these influence the work of everyday living and the health of the individual, including their capacity to respond to illness.

As I have described, being aware of these wider determinants of health for daily living is not intended to extend the responsibility or reach of medical practice; but rather the opposite. Illich (1973) warned about the dangers of overmedicalisation of (all aspects) of health. He described the iatrogenic harm that could result from using medicine and medical practice to try and control ever wider determinants of health. Today, we see a growing literature on the harms to individuals being created by too much medicine – too much screening, too much testing and overextension of medical diagnosis to describe wider societal problems. Optimising medical care has become the end point of healthcare. We strive to see people, diagnose people and start treatment – all as quickly as we can and with limited reference to a broader end point of health for daily living. Medicine has become an end in itself; rather than a means to an end – communities are better able to manage health for daily living. Just as Illich predicted, medicine is becoming part of the problem – contributing to the tsunami of healthcare needs facing today's patients and healthcare systems.

The WHO described this approach within Western medicine as the command and control of disease. Whilst a potentially appropriate and valuable approach for managing acute illness such as outbreaks of infection, authors have challenged its usefulness in managing the newly emerging problems of chronic illness and multimorbidity (see Tinetti and Fried 2004). Within a command and control approach, for an individual living with multiple long-term conditions, best care is achieved by efficient, coordinated management of each of those individual diseases. But Hughes et al. (2013) highlighted the limitations of this approach in a critique of guideline care. They used an example of a fictitious patient, Alice, living with five common long-term conditions (diabetes, cardiovascular disease, osteoarthritis, depression and chronic obstructive pulmonary disease). They listed what Alice's 'best' care would look like if each of the guidelines for these conditions was optimally applied. Alice ends up on over 11 medicines a day, attending ten follow-up appointments, being asked to do nine self-care activities, all on top of her usual daily routines. Medical care may improve the control of her diseases, but may also come at the cost of reducing her capacity for daily living. In this scenario, medicine has become an end in itself, rather than a means to a broader end. This problem is replicated in communities and healthcare settings across the world.

In the last couple of decades, a number of authors have started to describe, define and challenge the burden placed on patients by treatment plans focused on optimising disease care. In her work on living after a stroke, Gallacher (2018) argues that we need to focus more on the everyday work experienced by people living with long term conditions. This work includes the pre-existing everyday work that a person does to keep a roof over their head, food on the table and to support family and friends. Add to that the work of living with an illness, for example, disability following a stroke, as well as the treatment work created by healthcare, on the lines described for Alice. From all of this, we start to see quite a different view of the 'value' of healthcare.

May et al. (2009) proposed that we need to recognise a new approach for healthcare – what they described as Minimally Disruptive Medicine. Since then, they have described the Burden of Treatment Theory – shining a light on the work that patients do to manage everyday illness and associated healthcare in order to inform new ways of thinking about healthcare (May et al. 2014). From this, they have described and tested a tool to measure Treatment Burden, to help healthcare professionals recognise, address and monitor this important impact of care (Tran et al. 2012). Other teams have developed and validated tools for use in specific circumstances, for example multimorbidity (Duncan et al. 2018). This body of work serves to recognise and highlight the significance of a previously under-recognised impact of condition-focused (specialist) healthcare and so highlight the need to strengthen whole person generalist approaches.

So we need to reset the goals of healthcare. By shifting our focus from optimising disease control, to optimising the work of daily living, we recognise that healthcare happens in the context of people's daily lives. And this needs to be factored in to the way we describe and set goals for healthcare. Our goals for healthcare need to focus on the work that people do, rather than just the disease process they have. This needs fundamental changes in the focus, priorities and actions of healthcare delivery, including in how we recognise and judge good care. So how do we do that in practice? Let's take a look.

1.4   THE WORK OF WHOLE PERSON MEDICINE: CREATING UNDERSTANDING IN CONTEXT

Achieving a goal of supporting health for daily living relies on us understanding an individual in context, so that we can consider the potential value and harm of medical care in supporting health for daily living. Creating tailored, individualised understanding of illness and the value or place of medicalisation of illness in context is the distinct work of the advanced medical generalist. This work uses skills to critically explore, explain and evaluate individual illness experience. Guidelines inform each stage of the work, but they do not dictate the outcome. The generalist practitioner uses the knowledge of guidelines but goes further to create new understanding of illness for this individual in their context. This work to tailor care to the individual and context is the knowledge work of advanced generalist practice. It is a distinct and different way of doing medical practice.

Therefore, I recognise generalist practitioners as knowledge workers – people who 'think for a living' (Drucker 1959). Knowledge workers can be found in many different work settings, not just healthcare. In most industries, they are valued for their abilities to undertake 'non-routine problem solving'; using an 'abstract knowledge base to [creatively] complete tasks, [adapting] the specific response to the context'. Knowledge workers are not unique to healthcare but are found in many different workplaces. Their distinct skills and expertise lies in their ability to use knowledge critically and creatively to provide an adaptive response to complex problems (see https://en.wikipedia.org/wiki/Knowledge_worker for further discussion).

Applied evidence-based medicine (EBM) is also a form of knowledge work. EBM applied the principles of hypothetico-deductive reasoning and the knowledge derived from biomedical research to describe the probability that a patient has a named condition (generate a diagnosis) and would therefore benefit from treatment (describe a treatment plan). Advanced generalist practice is grounded in scientific knowledge practice, but uses a different model of clinical reasoning and an extended evidence base in order to generate an understanding of whole person illness to support a management plan (Reeve 2010, Interpretive Medicine). Yet, it uses a form of scientific reasoning that is not routinely taught in health professional training. If we want to deliver whole person medicine, we will need to address that gap. This will be the focus of my discussion in Chapter 2.

1.5 THE CONTEXT OF WHOLE PERSON MEDICINE: COMPLEX INTERVENTIONS

My fifth principle for understanding whole person, generalist care recognises that all of this work doesn't happen in a vacuum. The generalist physician who seeks to understand their patient in context – the individual and their illness – does so in the context of a healthcare system which shapes and drives the work they do.

My research has repeatedly highlighted that health professionals experience a number of barriers to delivering whole person tailored care in their everyday workplace. This includes a perceived lack of permission to tailor care; a failure to prioritise this complex work in the array of competing pressures on healthcare professionals; a lack of skills, confidence and resources to support the work; and a lack of feedback to support continuing practice. These are significant blocks that must be addressed if we are to deliver whole person, generalist care, now. Meaning we must not only change the training of professionals but also the contexts in which they work.

Tailoring healthcare to individual circumstances is an example of what is described as a 'wicked problem'. A wicked problem is one that can't be 'solved' or 'fixed' because there is no one single solution, and because the situation is constantly changing. Here, wicked doesn't mean 'bad' but instead refers to a problem that resists a simple or straightforward solution. Making individually tailored decisions about healthcare needs can be seen as a wicked problem. Understanding whole person illness requires us to consider the interplay of illness and pathology, in the context of a creative self supported (or otherwise) by multiple factors, and living their daily life in the context of many interacting elements. All of these elements interact and shape the individual experience of illness, and so the tailored intervention needed to help. Therefore, we need a healthcare system which can be flexible, adapting to context in making decisions about what to do, and what outcomes can be expected. Yet, our current disease-focused model of healthcare is a more linear model – describing pathways for assessment, diagnosis, management and monitoring of healthcare. To support generalist healthcare, we need to shift to a model that supports 'complex interventions'.

A complex intervention has multiple component parts, giving it the flexibility to adapt to variation in individuals and contexts. But a complex intervention is not a 'free for all'. It will have defined constant elements that make the model of care distinct, and also variable elements that make it flexible for context (McPherson and Schroer 2007). In generalist healthcare, the constant component is the knowledge work of whole person medicine – the distinct element that contrasts the approach with specialist disease-focused care. The variable components will depend on circumstances and context. They may include the data available to support decision making, the skills and make up of clinical teams available to assess individual needs and the community resources including social prescribing, available to support management.

I'll go into all of this in more detail in the next chapter, but let me briefly illustrate with a (fictitious) case example. Imran is a husband and grandfather who also has a busy role as a member of his local community group and who has developed memory loss and diabetes. If we just focus on his medical conditions – dementia and diabetes – there are clear rules and paths of care to follow that tell us about his diagnosis and his medical management. But if we factor in the issues we have discussed in this chapter, then things change. The dementia and diabetes are two elements in the broader work of daily living for Imran. Thinking about Imran's creative capacity, there are some stable elements supporting this daily work (the input from his family and family roles) but also some variable elements (the struggle with maintaining support for his local community group). Factoring in some new 'work' – managing his medical conditions – puts additional pressure on this delicate balance. And then Imran's wife dies unexpectedly. Even in this simplified case, it is clear that there is no one definition of best care for Imran. Tailored generalist care, will require negotiating and creating a best understanding in context for Imran now. We will need to follow-up and review how the plan is working for Imran, and potentially change it if it's not helping his health for daily living. And when life throws in something unexpected, we will need to be ready to review and revise everything. Tailored care to manage wicked problems needs to be flexible and adaptable in its delivery – requiring the knowledge work expertise of clinicians trained in advanced generalist practice. Wicked problems need to be managed in complex healthcare systems. Disease-focused healthcare systems are designed to offer linear pathways of care for a patient. I will discuss the implications for redesign of our healthcare systems in later chapters.

1.6 SUMMARY

In this chapter, I have outlined the five principles of expert generalist practice.

1. The *purpose* for the generalist, whole person medicine – creating a whole person understanding of illness.
2. The *focus* for whole person medicine – understanding the person we care for.
3. The *goal* of whole person medicine – enhancing health as a resource people need for daily living.
4. The *work* of whole person medicine – the wisdom of understanding in context.
5. The *context* in which generalist medicine happens – delivering a complex intervention in a healthcare setting designed to support this work.

The golden thread through these principles is the individual. The clinical professions have long recognised that our patients – the individuals we work with – drive *why* we do the work we do. Now, we must recognise that the person needs to define *how* we work too.

The task of whole person medicine is being to enable and enhance the creative capacity of that individual to live their daily life. This task to explore, explain and evaluate tailored interpretations of illness, is a task that requires the skills of the distinct knowledge work of advanced generalist practice. In this chapter, I have outlined why we need to shift the understanding of our professional role from a focus on what we know, to a new focus on how we use what we know to support our patients (Wenzel 2017).

This is the work of the advanced generalist practitioner to create, use and critique new understanding (or knowledge-in-context) about a complex problem. It is a form of scientific knowledge work that goes beyond the traditional descriptions of medical practice described by condition-specific specialist healthcare. In the next chapter, I will explore in more depth how we do this work.

REFERENCES

Bury M. (1982). Chronic illness as biographical disruption. Sociology of Health & Illness, 4(2), pp. 167–182.

Carel H. (2008). Illness (The Art of Living). Oxon: Routledge.

Dahlgren G, Whitehead M. (1991). Policies and Strategies to Promote Social Equity in Health. Stockholm, Sweden: Institute for Futures Studies.

Dowrick C. (Ed). (2019). Person-Centred Primary Care. Searching for the Self. Oxon: Routledge.

Drucker P. (1959). The Landmarks of Tomorrow. London: Routledge.

Duncan P et al. (2018). Development and validation of the multimorbidity treatment burden questionnaire (MTBQ). BMJ Open 8(4), p. e019413.

Faircloth CA, Boylstein C, Rittman M, Young ME, Gubrium J. (2004). Sudden illness and biographical flow in narratives of stroke recovery. Sociology of Health & Illness, 26(2), pp. 242–261.

Gallacher K et al. (2013). Uncovering treatment burden as a key concept for stroke care: A systematic review of qualitative literature. PLoS Med, 10, p. e1001473.

Griffiths J. (2016). Choosing to be a jack of all trades. https://www.youtube.com/watch?v=-BfcvI49GCw

Harden B. (2017). Person-centred approaches: Empowering people in their lives and communities to enable an upgrade in prevention, wellbeing, health care and support. Health Education England. https://www.skillsforhealth.org.uk/info-hub/person-centred-approaches-2017/

Howe A. (2012). Medical Generalism. Why Expertise in Whole Person Medicine Matters. Royal College of General Practitioners.

Hughes L, McMurdo MET, Guthrie B. (2013). Guidelines for people not diseases: The challenges of applying UK clinical guidelines to people with multimorbidity. Age Aging, 42, pp. 62–69.

Illich I. (1973). Limits to Medicine: Medical Nemesis – the Expropriation of Health. Penguin Books.

Lewis S. (2013). The two faces of generalism. Journal of Health Services Policy and Research, 19, pp. 1–2.

Maslow AH. (1943). A theory of human motivation. Psychological Review, 50, pp. 370–396.

May CR et al. (2009). We need minimally disruptive medicine. BMJ, 339, p. b2803.

May CR et al. (2014). Rethinking the patient: Using the burden of treatment theory to understand the changing dynamics of illness. BMC Health Services Research, 14, p. 281.

McPherson H, Schroer S (2007). Acupuncture as a complex intervention for depression: A consensus method to develop a standardised treatment protocol for a randomised controlled trial. Complementary Therapies in Medicine, 15, pp. 92–100.

Reeve J. (2006). Understanding distress in people with terminal cancer: The role of the general practitioner. PhD thesis, University of Liverpool, Liverpool.

Reeve J (2010). Interpretive medicine: Supporting generalism in a changing primary care world. Occasional Paper Series Royal College of General Practitioners, 88, pp. 1–20.

Reeve J. (2019). Unlocking the creative capacity of the self. In Dowrick C (Ed). Person-Centred Primary Care. Searching for the Self. Oxon: Routledge.

Reeve J, Lynch T, Lloyd-Williams M, Payne S (2012). From personal challenge to technical fix: The risks of depersonalised care. Health and Social Care in the Community, 20(2), pp. 145–154.

Tinetti ME, Fried T (2004). The end of a disease era. American Journal of Medicine, 116, pp. 179–185.

Tran VT et al. (2012). Development and description of measurement properties of an instrument to assess treatment burden among patients with multiple chronic conditions. BMC Medicine, 10, p. 68.

Williams G. (1984). The genesis of chronic illness: Narrative reconstruction. Sociology of Health & Illness, 6(2), pp. 175–200.

Williams SJ. (2000). Chronic illness as biographical disruption or biographical disruption as chronic illness? Reflections on a core concept. Sociology of Health & Illness, 22(1), pp. 40–67.

Williamson DL, Carr J. (2009). Health as a resource for everyday life: Advancing the conceptualisation. Critical Public Health, 19, pp. 107–122.

World Health Organization (WHO). (1986). Ottawa Charter for Health Promotion. World Health Organization.

CHAPTER 2

Wise foundations: The knowledge work of practice

....

In Chapter 1, I outlined the principles of whole person medicine and introduced why we need to recognise the knowledge work at the core of advanced generalist practice. In this chapter, I explore what knowledge work is and how generalist knowledge work differs from the knowledge work of specialist healthcare.

2.1 THE KNOWLEDGE WORK OF CLINICAL PRACTICE

People see clinicians when they have a problem with their health. The clinician's job is to understand the problem, help find a way to deal with it and (ideally) put plans in place to check things are getting better. This is the knowledge work of clinical practice – the way we create, use and learn from knowledge in everyday practice.

We don't often hear people (patients or professionals) talking about the knowledge *work* of clinical practice. Instead, people talk about what their doctor knows. Patients may describe, 'my doctor knows all about me'. A specialist will be respected for knowing 'everything' about their field of medicine. In the past, we defined a profession by the 'body of knowledge' that it owned and needed to do its job (Scambler 2018). It is much more common to describe medical practice in terms of what we know.

But in 2017, Richard Wenzel, writing in the *New England Journal of Medicine*, proposed that modern clinical practice should not be defined by what we know but by how we use what we know to achieve a defined goal. Wenzel described that we live in a world of competing facts, ideas

DOI: 10.1201/9781003297222-2

and perspectives about health and illness. To deal with this, he argued that we need to focus not just on the knowledge itself but also on the practice of the person using that knowledge. Rather than defining best practice by the knowledge we use (good or bad, right or wrong), he suggested that we understand best practice in terms of the way that the clinician uses knowledge in practice. He argued that clinicians need three things to support this knowledge work: curiosity, clarity and critical thinking. He proposed that medical education needs to help clinicians not only acquire knowledge but also develop the skills needed to use it wisely (Wenzel 2017). So how does current medical practice support curiosity, clarity and critical thinking?

2.2 THE KNOWLEDGE WORK OF SPECIALIST MEDICINE

We don't commonly use the phrase 'knowledge work' when we talk about medicine, but we do train practitioners in the work of knowledge management. I start this chapter by looking at how we currently do that.

Modern healthcare defines best practice as practice-based-on-evidence. Therefore, what we define as *good evidence* shapes our understanding of what is *best practice*. As I have already described, our current understanding of best evidence is grounded in the principles of evidence-based medicine (EBM). EBM was originally developed as a tool to support life-long professional learning – to help practitioners to find and critique new scientific research evidence and so decide whether and how to use it in practice. David Sackett is widely acknowledged as the pioneer of EBM. Now retired, he was a general internist and clinical epidemiologist working in Canada. The principles of clinical epidemiology – 'the investigation and control of the distribution and determinants of *disease*' [my emphasis] underpin the assumptions of EBM (Sackett et al. 1991). Therefore, EBM was designed to support the knowledge work of *disease-focused* medical practice. And that matters because it shapes the way we currently practice medicine, including the knowledge work that we do.

EBM defined a *hierarchy* of evidence for practitioners to consider when making clinical judgements about the use of knowledge in practice (Figure 2.1). This hierarchy defined the trustworthiness of evidence for clinical decision making based on the scientific method used to produce the knowledge (see Box 2.1). Best evidence, from an EBM perspective, is that derived from experimental scientific methods – randomised trials and syntheses of those studies. Best practice becomes defined by and synonymous with the experimental method used in clinical trials – namely hypothetico-deductive reasoning.

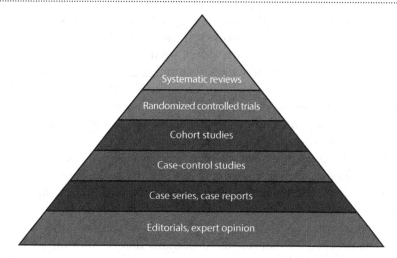

Figure 2.1 The hierarchy of evidence described by EBM.

BOX 2.1 THE EBM HIERARCHY OF KNOWLEDGE

EBM described a hierarchy of 'best' knowledge for clinical practice – encouraging clinicians to value the insights gained from experimental research studies above any other.

Research studies describing the biographical impact of illness such as diabetes on daily living (see Chapter 1) would be considered of less value than a randomised clinical trial in guiding clinical management.

Some EBM accounts describe an additional top layer in the hierarchy – the 'n of 1 trial'. This view recognises that the best knowledge we can have about a treatment for a patient is the knowledge we gain when we try out the treatment on that individual – the knowledge we gain from an applied form of 'whole person medicine'. This approach makes 'clinical judgement' of the efficacy of a treatment for an individual (whole person) the highest form of evidence in EBM. However, none of these accounts have adequately described how this form of 'clinical judgement' can be distinguished from the category of 'expert opinion' which appears at the bottom of the hierarchy. In practice, we therefore fail to recognise and value this practice of whole person medicine.

The hierarchy of evidence ranks the quality and trustworthiness of evidence (or knowledge) used in clinical decision making according to the methodological approach used to generate it. EBM is grounded in a hypothetico-deductive scientific framework and so values evidence generated using these methods above other forms of evidence.

Such methods are well suited to the study of defined disease states that can be objectively and consistently measured. Take the example of diabetes. It is possible to clearly define what diabetes is, and so objectively assess if someone has the condition, and if a treatment makes that condition better or worse. In the clinical setting, if we want to know about the best ways to manage diabetes, we should use knowledge derived from experimental study designs such as clinical trials to give us an objective assessment of the benefit of a treatment.

This can be helpful when a patient presents with a defined disease state, preferably just the one disease and ideally something acute. For example, John is 22 years old and comes to see me with a three-day worsening sore throat. He wants to know if he has a streptococcal infection and whether he needs antibiotics. He has enlarged tonsils with visible pus present. We can test the hypothesis that he does indeed have strep throat by applying the Centor criteria. He scores 4, meaning he has a 30–60% chance of having streptococcal infection. The evidence base suggests that antibiotics will shorten the duration of his illness by about a day with a small reduction in the small absolute risk of developing complications from the infection (NICE 2018). John feels the benefit outweighs the risks of antibiotic use and requests a prescription.

But in my daily practice, it is increasingly rare to see a problem like John's. As an experienced GP in the practice, I am much more likely to see people with symptoms related to multiple interacting long-term conditions, or with persisting symptoms with no underlying disease identified. Applying a hypothetico-deductive model of clinical reasoning to someone who doesn't have a single disease process behind their illness presentation is likely to cause problems for us both.

Take, for example, the case of Ibrahim. He comes to see me because he is feeling tired all the time. He has been talking with friends and wonders if he might have developed diabetes. There are externally defined criteria for diabetes so we can use a hypothetico-deductive approach to test Ibrahim's idea. I collect data from a history, examination and blood tests to use to test a hypothesis (assess the likelihood) that Ibrahim has diabetes. We get his test results back and find that Ibrahim doesn't meet the criteria for a diagnosis of diabetes. This model of practice has made sure I don't inappropriately start Ibrahim on a course of treatment that he won't benefit from. But it hasn't helped Ibrahim, or me, to get to the bottom of the problem. So what do we do next?

We could generate a whole new set of hypotheses (e.g., underactive thyroid, anaemia) and collect more data (blood tests) to test them (Henegan et al. 2009). Indeed, this is a common approach we see in practice and perhaps gives us an idea of why we are seeing escalating levels of testing in current medical practice. Hypothetico-deductive testing is a very inefficient form of clinical practice in the primary care setting where patients present undifferentiated, and often whole person, health needs (Müskens et al. 2022). But this approach will also miss the non-disease–related factors contributing to Ibrahim's symptoms – including the work of daily living, and issues related to creative capacity that I discussed in Chapter 1. If we fail to recognise and understand the impact of these wider issues on Ibrahim's experience of tiredness, we risk entering a recurrent cycle of inappropriate medicalisation of his illness – repeated disease testing and even trial of treatments which are at best unhelpful, and at worse distract from the search for effective ways forward.

If we want to create a tailored, whole person understanding of illness in context, disease-focused experimental study designs may not be the best way to generate the knowledge we need for practice. We need to rethink our approach to the use of knowledge in practice.

2.3 THE ALTERNATIVE KNOWLEDGE WORK OF GENERALIST PRACTICE

We now have a small, but growing, body of research that describes how primary care practitioners create tailored whole person understanding of illness. This describes that the knowledge work of whole person primary care is different to the condition-specific specialist approach, and in two important ways: firstly, it is based on inductive (not deductive) reasoning, and secondly, it relies on knowledge generated in practice. Let's consider each in turn.

Inductive foraging

Specialist practice is built on a principle of hypothetico-deductive reasoning. We start with a question: What is wrong with this person? To explore and answer that questions, we use an externally developed and defined body of knowledge as a reference point. Take the example of a defined disease state such as a cataract. Hypothetico-deductive reasoning gives us an objective and certain starting point – we know with certainty that cataracts exist and what they are. In the clinical setting, we may generate a hypothesis that our patient has a cataract. This allows us to objectively test a patient's illness against this reference point to decide (deduce) if they do, or don't, have that condition (a cataract) and so are likely to benefit from treatment. If our original starting point is true (cataracts really exist), and we have robustly and objectively tested our hypothesis, then it must be true that this person has cataracts.

Generalist practice uses a different approach. Donner Banzhoff is a German academic GP whose team has observed generalist consultations over many years. Based on this work, he argues that in seeking to 'fit' patients to a defined disease process using the hypothetico-deductive approach, we may miss important information (Donner-Banzhoff and Hertwig 2014). For example, he discusses the clinician who uses the PHQ9 (a tool to assess risk of depression) to assess a person presenting in distress. The PHQ9 tool may indicate the individual meets the threshold for moderate depression and so (according to stepped care) should be recommended an antidepressant. But in following this path, the clinician may have missed out the opportunity to explore this distress further, and in doing so discover that this individual is also dealing with the trauma of bereavement and would potentially benefit from other approaches. It is increasingly uncommon for us to see patients with a single condition causing their illness experience. It is because of this that Donner-Banzhoff has criticised the hypothetico-deductive model for generalist practice because of the risk of what he describes as 'premature closure'.

Instead, he has described the exploratory work that generalist clinicians do to understand whole person illness. He called this inductive foraging. In a consultation, the generalist clinician 'goes looking' – seeking to understand an individual's illness *in context*. They explore the multiple factors that may contribute to, and so help explain, the illness that a person has presented. The generalist clinician uses an inductive reasoning process to explore and generate a whole person understanding (or so-called probable explanation) of illness based on these observations. Donner-Banzhoff argued that this approach improves what he called the 'diagnostic yield' of practice. It also allows the clinician to generate an internally developed set of hypotheses that then allow a more focused exploration and testing.

I'll come back to inductive reasoning again shortly, but the key element this work raises is in recognising a different form of knowledge work for the generalist practitioner. Generalist practice doesn't just use external (disease) knowledge as a reference point to assess a patient's illness so that we can say whether they do or don't have that disease. Instead, practice involves the critical creation of a whole person explanation of that illness – the work of creating knowledge in context.

Generation of practice-based evidence: Gabbay and le May

This critical creative view of the knowledge work of clinical practice is also recognised and described in the work of Gabbay and le May. They spent extended periods of time in the general practice setting observing the work that clinicians do to make sense of illness in practice. Their findings propose that clinicians engaged in whole person care work to create what they called knowledge-in-practice-in-context or practice-based evidence (Gabbay and le May 2011, 2023).

Gabbay and le May's work draws on research into knowledge work practice conducted outside of the healthcare setting. Nonaka and Takeuchi (1995) studied the work of employees in Japanese companies who were engaged in managing complex problems. They recognised that workers cannot simply use objective, external facts to manage in-practice, complex problems. Instead, workers need to use both this established knowledge (external references) and also their own experiential knowledge (internal, in-practice understanding) in order to make sense of and manage complex, changing problems on the ground. Gabbay and le May observed clinicians in practice using similar approaches to manage the complex problems of whole person healthcare. They therefore set out to describe how clinicians do the work to find, create, use and critique knowledge-in-practice.

Based on their studies in the Japanese setting, Nonaka and Takeuchi (1995) developed a model to describe the knowledge work of everyday practice. They recognised four processes involved in acquiring and generating knowledge for practice, which they described as the SECI cycle. These are described in Box 2.2.

Gabbay and le May used these principles to critically examine their observations of knowledge work in general practice. They repeatedly saw that practitoners did not use the linear, hypothetico-deductive reasoning associated with applied EBM. Instead, practitioners used a wide variety of knowledge sources to explore and understand the clinical (and practice-level) problems of their everyday work. Practitioners were engaged in a dynamic, and cyclical, process of knowledge work – creating, using and critiquing knowledge in practice in context. External evidence (including guidelines for clinical care) was used as a knowledge source, but did not dictate practice. It was one source used in the inductive process of gathering information (on the lines described by Donner-Banzhoff) and critically examining it in order to create a new understanding of the problem in context. Gabbay and le May's observations also encourage us to rethink our assumptions about clinical reasoning for practice.

BOX 2.2 DESCRIBING THE FOUR
COMPONENTS OF THE SECI CYCLE

Socialisation describes an 'apprenticeship' stage of knowledge work. It involves workers (especially those new to practice) observing and imitating the practice of others in order to gain understanding and to share tacit knowledge. *The new GP trainee observing how different members of the team work as part of their practice induction is engaged in Socialisation.*

Externalisation occurs as the knowledge worker gains confidence and understanding in their work. The worker uses existing theory and knowledge to help them observe and explore, and so develop new knowledge in context. They start to test that knowledge by sharing it with others so that they can comment. *The GP trainee starts to test out their understanding in conversations with their trainer at team meetings. They may draw on Royal College of GPs and General Medical Council definitions of best practice to help them critically appraise what they are observing, developing and describing.*

Combination describes the developing knowledge a worker acquires, combines and modifies their growing sources of knowledge for practice – including external, objective evidence for practice and the internal knowledge generated through collective action. And so creates a new more sophisticated understanding of everyday practice. *The GP trainee integrates their knowledge of guidelines for best specialist care with their observation of best generalist care, and their experience of working with patients to start to generate their own deeper understanding of the expertise of whole person medical care.*

Internalisation is when this new knowledge becomes 'tacit' again – embedded in the 'internal working knowledge' of the professional. *The GP, over a lifetime of practice, becomes more comfortable with the complexities of everyday practice, the 'routine' generation of knowledge in practice in context and so the work of advanced generalist practice.*

Clinical reasoning refers to the processes by which clinicians collect, process and interpret patient information in order to guide decision making. Currently, medical practice recognises two approaches known as Type 1 (intuitive) and Type 2 (rational) reasoning (Croskerry 2009; see Box 2.3). Type 2 reasoning refers to the hypothetico-deductive

---

BOX 2.3 MODELS OF CLINICAL REASONING

There are two current models (Croskerry 2009):

Type 1 (intuitive) processes are very fast – used by experts most of the time.

Type 2 (rational – hypothetico-deductive) processes are slower, deliberate and more reliable and focus more on hypothesis and deductive clinical reasoning.

In this chapter, I propose we need to add a third model of clinical reasoning:

Type 3 (inductive) critical creation of new understanding based on inductive reasoning.

---

reasoning I have previously discussed. As we gain confidence in our clinical practice, we may start to revert to using the Type 1, intuitive logic that is sometimes referred to as pattern recognition. As a clinicians sees more cases of a particular problem, they start to recognise patterns in how people present, and can be managed. The experienced clinician creates so-called internal 'illness scripts' that guide quick

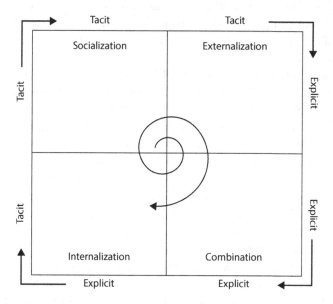

Figure 2.2   The SECI model of knowledge dimensions. Describing the creation of knowledge in context. (By Ibmgroup – Using an image editor, CC BY-SA 3.0, https://commons.wikimedia.org/w/index.php?curid=18653983.)

thinking, especially if we're dealing with a 'straightforward' case. If a clinician sees a patient who fits one of these internally held scripts, or patterns, they may bypass the full hypothetico-deductive approach and jump straight to a trial of treatment. For example, the cardiologist who has seen many cases of ischaemic heart disease recognises the 'characteristic features' and starts treatment even before they have completed an exercise stress test. Type 1 logic is seen as the 'shortcut' of the expert (their 'gut instinct'); however, it is the form of clinical reasoning most open to error (in terms of creating a wrong diagnosis). Type 2 is the 'gold standard' for clinical practice.

The work described by both Gabbay and le May and Donner-Banzhoff reveals clinicians doing a different type of knowledge work based on inductive practice. We therefore now need to recognise a third type of clinical reasoning – inductive reasoning.

In my own research, generalist clinicians have repeatedly told me they use their 'gut instinct' to support whole person care. This happens particularly when they identify patients whose clinical needs require something beyond guideline, or disease-focused, care. In my experience, many of these clinicians do not have a language to readily describe the complex (Type 3) knowledge work that they are doing, and so instead refer to it as using their 'gut instinct' or 'tacit knowledge'. The risk is that people conflate complex inductive practice with Type 1 intuitive reasoning – the 'silver' to the gold practice of Type 2 reasoning, and one that may be seen as only suitable for the most experienced practitioners.

Again, Gabbay and le May's work helps us here. They describe how clinicians use inductive approaches to generate new 'internal scripts' or patterns that can help with the pace and change of everyday practice. These they described as 'mindlines'. Mindlines are locally (and commonly tacitly) generated guidelines-for-practice, or practice-based evidence. Gabbay and le May's observations show how generalist clinicians use these knowledge work skills and the mindlines generated to help them manage complex clinical problems, adapt to change and continue to improve. Mindlines can therefore be used to support Type 1 (intuitive) clinical reasoning for everyday practice; but they are distinct from the disease-focused scripts used by specialist clinicians.

So the knowledge work of advanced generalist practice uses inductive practice to generate new knowledge in context to support whole person clinical care. The expertise of the advanced generalist practitoner is defined not by what they know (a little bit about a lot), but how they find and use knowledge to make sense of and manage whole person illness in context. Generalist practice is an advanced form of knowledge work for clinical practice – certainly no 'jack of all trades, master of none'.

Gabbay and le May described that clinicians most commonly learn these skills through apprenticeship – rooted in early training; and adapted, refined and reinforced by experience, training, peer learning and the impact of external pressures. They describe this as the development of contextual adroitness – the skills and confidence to transform information gained from patients, context and guidelines into the knowledge-in-practice-in-context for everyday working. Gabbay and le May focused on the work of GPs. In their latest book, fellow researchers describe how allied health professionals are also active in this process (Gabbay and le May 2023). Yet, my own research has revealed that many clinicians working in primary care do not feel confident in this form of clinical practice. So I now want to turn to think about how we can address that problem.

Defining a new model of knowledge work for everyday clinical practice

Based on my exploration of the knowledge work of advanced generalist practice so far, I now want to recognise and address three things. Firstly, I have described that we are dealing with a different scientific model of clinical practice – inductive over deductive reasoning. I will look in more detail about what that means for practice. Secondly, I have described that generalist practice uses a different point of reference to specialist medicine: one that is based on an internally (contextually) generated understanding of illness in context, rather than an externally defined statement of what things are (e.g., a disease state). I will look at how we develop that contextual understanding. My third point recognises that this has implications for how we understand 'best' practice. Specialist practice, using an external disease-focused reference, readily describes best practice by whether our reasoning (and diagnosis) is right or wrong. Generalist practice uses a different type of knowledge work, but as I have outlined, this is no 'opinion-based medicine' – the whim of clinician and patient on the day. Instead it is an advanced form of practice, grounded in scientific methods, but using an inductive approach to reasoning, data collection and analysis. Generalist practice still has, and needs, a reference point for judging best practice, but it needs a different 'standard' to that used for specialist practice. This is the third element that I will consider in discussing how we can integrate these approaches into the practice setting.

2.4 BARRIERS TO GENERALISM IN ACTION

First, I want to look more closely at what we know about what stops clinicians from doing person-centred advanced generalist care. Understanding the barriers will help us develop ways to improve whole person care.

Over the last 10 years, I have repeatedly explored barriers to generalist practice. These studies have consistently highlighted the same four key factors – with only minor, although significant, changes that I will discuss. My research was built using an established model called Normalisation Process Theory (May 2015). That theory describes that if we want a way of working, in this case generalist practice, to become a routine part of everyday healthcare, then we need to have four elements in place (Figure 2.3). Generalist practice must make sense to practitioners; so that they can engage with and start to do the work. Clinicians must have the skills and resources they need to do the work and the monitoring of their work should support their practice. My research has repeatedly shown that all four elements are missing for generalist care.

In surveys with GPs, primary care professionals (including nurses and pharmacists) and medical students, I have repeatedly described four key barriers (Figure 2.3). Firstly, clinicians don't feel that they have *permission* to deliver whole person care. Person-centred care is described as an ideal in professional training, including for GPs. But staff describes that when working in front-line practice, they fear personal and medicolegal complaints if they deviate from guideline-driven clinical care. Person-centred care is therefore supported in theory but not practice.

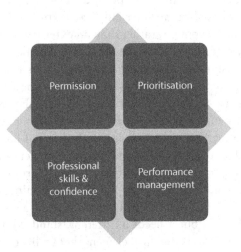

Figure 2.3   Four barriers to the actions of generalist practice in context.

Many staff described never having had any training in how to safely and effectively deliver whole person care. Others spoke of 'learning on the job' – an apprenticeship-type training that helped them understand how and why whole person care worked. But even those with the skills and confidence to use them described a lack of resources to support practice – for example, access to the data they needed for complex decisions. Therefore, people lack the *professional skills, confidence and resources* for the job.

The complex work of inductive practice is not *prioritised* in the design of a typical working day or week for professionals. In my early surveys, people described that they didn't have the time to do this complex work. Their comments supported calls for longer consultation times in primary care. More recently, this has changed. They now describe they don't have the 'headspace' for this work. Primary care clinicians are dealing with so many competing demands on their time (as they try to do 'a little about a lot') that they don't have the emotional and intellectual capacity for the inductive reasoning I discussed earlier in this chapter. As evermore tasks to do have been passed to general practice, clinicians simply don't have the capacity to undertake the more complex work. My research indicates that simply increasing consultation times may not be enough.

The fourth barrier to generalist knowledge work described is a lack of feedback needed to enable and encourage people to continue this complex work. At best, *performance management* processes ignore or overlook this complex form of practice. At worse, clinicians are criticised for not following a guideline. Clinicians therefore consistently describe that this work is not designed into their professional training, understanding and delivery of everyday professional practice.

So if we are to overcome these barriers, we need a new clear description of the knowledge work of advanced generalist practice providing permission for practice, designed into the training and organisation of practice, with a clear framework for recognising and rewarding best practice.

I will utilize case studies describing practice-based elements for each of these in the chapters that follow. But I start by looking at generalist knowledge work, and describing the 4Es that underpin best practice.

2.5 GENERALISM IN ACTION: THE 4Es OF BEST PRACTICE

In Chapter 1, I described that the goal of generalist medicine is to optimise health as a resource for daily living. To achieve this goal, we need to understand illness in context, recognising the multiple elements that contribute to both the whole person, individual experience of illness and so shaping options for management. We must work with patients to develop a tailored understanding of the problem and how to manage it.

In this chapter, I describe how tailored, generalist understanding of healthcare needs are different to disease-focused specialist understanding because it requires us to create an 'internal' reference point for our knowledge work. Specialist care works to assess if a patient meets (externally defined) criteria for a given disease, and so decide if they are 'eligible' for care. Generalist care works with individuals to create an internally developed, tailored understanding of their illness-in-context that both guides a plan for care and provides a reference point for monitoring the impact of care.

This doesn't mean that generalist care means clinicians should ignore evidence-based guidance on the diagnosis and management of disease. Guidelines and disease-based evidence are important sources of information for the generalist clinician to consider with their patients. They inform, but *do not dictate*, care. David Haslam, the Director of the key UK body which produces guidelines for NHS care, once described that clinicians should understand that NICE documents are 'guidelines not tramlines' (NICE 2018). Yet, as my research has shown, front-line clinicians repeatedly report feeling unconfident and unsupported in providing 'beyond guideline' care. The hypothetico-deductive reasoning of specialist medical care provides clinicians, and health systems, with a clear reference point against which to assess the quality of our care: whether we got the 'right' diagnosis or applied the correct management plan. We don't have an equivalent reference point for generalist (inductive) practice. So how can we know when we have done it well? We need a framework that describes the elements of best care so that we can train practitioners, design healthcare systems to deliver it and evaluate the impact of our healthcare.

Based on 20 years of studying the knowledge work of generalist medicine, I propose that best practice can be described by the 4Es: Epistemology, Exploration, Explanation and Evaluation.

To help me describe each of these, I'm going to use the example of Elsie. Elsie is a fictitious patient but based on people who I have seen over many years of clinical practice. Let me introduce you.

Elsie is an 80-year-old woman who has recently moved to supported accommodation. She has mild memory loss, no local family and wasn't coping at home. Her social worker arranged for her to move to her new home. Since she arrived, she stays in her room and doesn't talk with other residents or staff. The staff is worried that Elsie appears to be depressed and have asked you to visit. Elsie's clinical record in the practice shows that she is on a number of medicines, and is recorded as having a history of hypertension and underactive thyroid.

When we go to see Elsie, what are we trying to do? Based on our discussion so far, there are broadly two approaches we could take. We could use hypothetico-deductive reasoning to query whether Elsie has depression. I have previously described how Donner-Banzhoff warned us of the potential problems of this approach in shutting down our considerations too quickly. Alternatively, we could adopt a generalist, person-centred approach, and the principles of the 4Es to guide best practice. The 4Es describe the inductive knowledge work of generalist practice – including how do I know I have done it well (Epistemology) and the three elements needed to do the work (Explore, Explain and Evaluate). As I describe each of these in more detail, I will keep returning to Elsie's story to illustrate the ideas.

Epistemology: A framework for best generalist practice

Our goal in working with Elsie is to optimise her health for daily living. To do that, we need to create a tailored understanding of Elsie's health and illness in context, to guide our management plan. We will need to integrate many sources of information to create a new tailored understanding of Elsie's situation. This is the knowledge work of generalist practice. But how will we know if we have done that well? Here we must turn to the concepts of epistemology.

Epistemology is the theory of knowledge. It is fundamental to much of the science we use in everyday clinical practice, yet it is a concept that few of us encounter in regular clinical training. Epistemology is a branch of philosophy asking questions such as, how do we know what we know and – crucially for our current discussion – how can we trust what we know? Epistemology helps us to distinguish between opinion and justified belief (Watson n.d.).

There are many learned texts on epistemology (Coady and Chase 2019) that discuss the breadth and detail of discussions that have raged on this topic for centuries. Here, I want to focus on two key points to help us understand the difference between specialist and generalist best practice. Both relate to our understanding of truth.

Specialist science, and hypothetico-deductive reasoning, rely on the belief that we can objectively describe a 'true' answer about human illness. So, for example, there is a real or true disease state which we call coronary artery atheroma. We can objectively demonstrate that the arteries of the heart can become blocked by fatty deposits and that this alters the blood supply to heart muscle. Unblocking the arteries (objectively) improves the blood flow. We can be strongly confident that people with blocked arteries will have symptoms such as angina, and that these symptoms improve if we unblock the arteries. Our understanding of this 'truth' is built on objective, experimental scientific measurement and assessment of human hearts.

But not all disease, and certainly not all illness, can be described and explained using these approaches. Take, for example, the 'disease' that is depression. We don't (yet) have the detailed understanding of how the human body works to understand the mechanisms behind mood disorders in the same way as we can describe blocked coronary arteries. But people around the world also have different ways of understanding the experience of low mood. What Western medicine might describe as a pathological (disease) called 'depression' is understood differently in other cultures. For example, mood 'disorders' known as depression in the West were understood in Latvia as a collective social experience of oppression (Skultans 2003). My intention is not to debate the 'true' meaning of depression, but rather to recognise that what we believe or understand to be 'true' depends on the perspective from which we look (see, for example, Seale and Pattison 2001).

Therefore, truth depends on the perspective from which we look. But that doesn't mean that we can't judge between different (and potentially competing) concepts of truth. The philosophy of epistemology, and the scientific practice developed from it, provides us with frameworks by which we can judge the truth or trustworthiness of competing knowledge. For hypothetico-deductive reasoning, we have the principles embedded in clinical epidemiology and statistical method to support us. We use this to help us recognise, address and hopefully avoid unacceptable variation in care. But there are also frameworks that we can use in assessing the inductive reasoning we need for the complexity of whole person practice. It is possible to describe criteria that help us to differentiate between 'opinion' and 'justified belief', and so to differentiate between practice that is rigorous and robust, or inadequate.

In 2010, I described an epistemological framework for best practice in inductive, advanced generalist practice in what I described as a model of Interpretive Medicine. My Wise framework translates established scientific research practice in inductive reasoning into the clinical context. The work described that if we want to be confident in

---

BOX 2.4 THE WISE FRAMEWORK – FIVE ELEMENTS OF BEST PRACTICE IN INTERPRETIVE MEDICINE

DATA COLLECTION We have collected all the data or information needed to fully explore and understand the illness. Including that we haven't prematurely shut down the conversation through hypothetico-deductive reasoning.

EXPLORATION We have explored all data sources (including patient's story, bio-medical/guideline data, and professional understanding of context) to understand how it relates to/helps us understand individual health for daily living.

EXPLANATION We have created a 'best' explanation of the illness that works for all parties – patient, practitioner and health system – and covers all the data sources.

CHECKING Safety netting – checking we haven't missed something, overlooked something or made inappropriate assumptions.

TRIAL & LEARN We have made a plan to follow-up, assess and potentially revise our understanding of the illness.

---

the knowledge we generate in practice in context, we need to establish and demonstrate good practice in five areas (Reeve 2010). These are described in Box 2.4.

I use this framework when teaching generalist epistemological principles. I'll share some of the feedback that I have received when I discuss the CATALYST programme in Chapter 4. But to start with, let's apply that framework to understand how we consult with Elsie.

Before I go and see Elsie, I look through her clinical records to understand – as far as I can – the history and context of her current healthcare. Obvious places to start include the coded list of conditions in her medical problem list and of course her medication list. I can see to what extent she has, or hasn't, been meeting guideline-described optimal management of her blood pressure and her thyroid function.

I meet Elsie in person to find out more about her daily living, her health, what she likes to do and what she is struggling with. Elsie mainly sits, and lies, on her bed as we talk. I get as much information from watching her interacting with me, staff and her still new home space as I do from what she tells me. I can also check some basic observations of her physical health. I talk with staff and other residents. There are no family and friends visiting. I think I've managed a comprehensive DATA COLLECTION, but I'm open to the idea that there is more to learn.

I EXPLORE all these elements with Elsie, with her carers, and with the clinical team back at the practice. How significant is each element in shaping Elsie's daily living? What do we still need to know – where are the gaps?

Together, we start to consider that Elsie's blood pressure tablets may be causing more harm than benefit. The EXPLANATION we are creating reflects the full range of data we have collected. For example, Elsie doesn't like taking tablets and her blood pressure is low end of normal, especially for an 80-year-old woman. Elsie's social isolation seems far more of a concern for daily living than any risk associated with hypertension, and we're worried that a low blood pressure may be holding Elsie back from everyday activities. We are thinking of stopping her hypertension medicines.

I talk things over at the practice frailty meeting. We consider whether we'd be thinking on the same lines if Elsie was 60, not 80; or if she had family members arguing that she should stay on the tablets. By CHECKING things over with clinical staff, carers and Elsie, we are making sure we haven't missed something.

So we decide to implement a TRIAL & LEARN approach – to stop Elsie's blood pressure tablets and observe whether we see any change, improvement even. We'll withdraw them gradually and the staff will help monitor her blood pressure. We plan to meet again to review the impact on daily living, with the option to revise the plan if needed.

Using the Wise framework, I can see that we have covered the five elements of good practice. My explanation is a structured and reasonable interpretation of the observations we have made. I have made plans to implement, review and, if necessary, revise the plan. This is beyond guideline care, but from a generalist perspective it is 'good' care. Do you agree?

I often use this example with students when we are discussing generalist practice. The (epistemological) framework provides a 'quality standard' for my assessment of Elsie's healthcare needs. The example also reveals the three main elements of knowledge work practice involved. Next, I want to look a bit closer at each of those.

Exploration: Inductive exploration

Exploration describes the process of collecting the information I need to create a tailored explanation. This is the inductive foraging described by Donner-Banzhoff and involves both the externalisation and combination

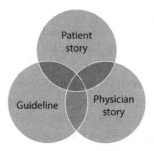

Figure 2.4 Data sources considered by clinicians during inductive exploration.

elements described in Gabbay and le May's account of the SECI process. Exploration takes place in a conversation with a patient such as Elsie; but also in consultation with case notes, published guidelines and evidence, conversations with local clinicians and services. It is an exploration, leading to the combination of stories from the patient (and carer/context), the physician (and team/local service) and the external evidence (guidelines) (Figure 2.4). These generalist conversations differ from the hypothetico-deductive conversations of specialist consultations. We can draw on scientific (research) practice to look more closely at how. We'll use Elsie again and think about how we understand her blood pressure.

In my account of Interpretive Medicine, I recognised that there are many similarities between interviews that take place in a clinical setting, and interviews for research. Both seek to help us understand something better. But as I described, the clinical interview method we teach tends to focus on hypothesis testing and so doesn't adequately support an exploratory, inductive approach.

In the research setting, Kvale has described two types of interviews used to generate the data and information we needed for knowledge generation (Kvale and Brinkmann, 2008). The first, he described as a 'mining' conversation. We use mining interviews in research that adopts a hypothetico-deductive approach. The researcher has a question which can be answered with a right or wrong answer. The purpose of a research interview is to extract the data we need to answer that question accurately. We can apply this same way of thinking to our clinical conversations with Elsie. If we take a hypothetico-deductive stance, our job is therefore to 'extract' the information we need from a conversation with Elsie to decide if she meets the diagnostic criteria. So our question is: Does Elsie have depression? A mining approach might use a structured tool such as PHQ9 to mine for, or extract, a series of data that help us to assess the probability that Elsie has depression. If this data suggests she does have depression, we may follow up with further focused questions to corroborate our hypothesis and to guide management (e.g., Has she ever been treated for depression before? Did she find antidepressants helpful?).

By contrast, Kvale described a second approach – that of a 'travelling' interview. Both people in this conversation are creating and shaping the information we are gathering to understand the problem. This is the model that best fits an inductive reasoning approach – whether in the research, or clinical context. A travelling interview with Elsie might start by exploring what she used to do before she came to live in the sheltered accommodation. Has that changed, and if so, why? Does she want to do anything about that? Travelling consultations require us to be curious and even potentially creative with our patients – to consider a wide range of factors that may link to an illness experience (including context and their creative capacity), and to reflect with our patients on if and how these experiences may related to the illness problem. Travelling consultations still require us to be critical and questioning as we look for patterns and anomalies in the information being generated, to consider gaps in what we're seeing and hearing, so that we can openly discuss and negotiate with our patients to create a tailored explanation or interpretation of their illness.

From the earliest stages of our clinical training, we are encouraged to listen to our patients: 'listen to your patient [s]he is telling you the diagnosis' (Bliss 1999). Using the idea of travelling, instead of mining, in our consultations helps to keep us actively listening, foraging and learning.

Explanation

It will already be apparent that the 4Es of generalist knowledge work are not discrete or linear. Through our exploration of Elsie's mood, we have been starting to create (and critically try out) possible explanations with Elsie. By exploring reasons why Elsie's daily living has changed – why she has become more subdued – we have been moving between explanation and exploration. A key aspect of this is to avoid the error we considered in type 1 reasoning – jumping to a premature conclusion about what is happening based on pattern recognition. By cycling between emerging ideas (explanations) and further exploration, we continue to explore and test our ideas. We use our epistemological framework to keep checking we haven't missed anything, jumped to conclusions, or overlooked an important factor (for example, Elsie telling us she used to have a dog but wasn't allowed to bring him to her new home ...).

Evaluation: Trial and learn

We use inductive reasoning to generate an explanation based on the observations and evidence we have available. (Indeed, this might even be better described as abductive reasoning – inference to the best explanation.) In both cases, our reasoning can be regarded as robust and trustworthy so long as we have followed the logic described within frameworks such as that of Interpretive Medicine. But our reasoning is inherently 'uncertain' because we are describing a complex and changing phenomenon. As described in Interpretive Medicine, the robustness or trustworthiness of inductive reasoning therefore relies on embedding a process of evaluation and learning into the interpretive, or decision-making, process. We assess the trustworthiness (justified belief) of interpretive knowledge, in part, by its capacity to predict and explain what follows.

Let's return to Elsie again to illustrate this point. Based on our whole person exploration, we have created an explanation with Elsie and her carers that she is overmedicalised. Instead of managing her risk and disease profile, her medication regime is burdening Elsie and slowing her down. Her blood pressure is too low, and her thyroid medication seems to leaving her with less energy too. We agree to try reducing some of Elsie's medicines and plan to actively follow-up with Elsie in a month's time to assess whether the changes have made any difference. Mainly, we want to check that there hasn't been any harm – benefits may take a little longer to show.

I stop her blood pressure medicines and return in a month. When I return, I find a different Elsie. She is up and about, interacting with staff and residents. Her personality is starting to shine through – and she can be quite grumpy at times! But the staff much prefer a 'grumpy Elsie' to the quiet and isolated Elsie of previously. Elsie's blood pressure is now 'off target' from a guideline perspective, but her health for daily living is much improved. We agree this is a 'compromise' worth making (Kings Fund 2013).

This example illustrates the importance and value of continuity in advanced generalist practice. Many have voiced concerns that continuity of care is being designed out of primary care practice in the UK, with a negative impact on satisfaction for patient and professionals alike. But we can also see that a failure to design maintenance of continuity into primary care practice has a potentially significant impact on the quality and safety of care. Continuity matters not (just) because of its impact on relationships and patient satisfaction, but also because it allows the clinician to review the utility of knowledge generated in context and, if appropriate, amend it in light of the new observations. Capacity for this 'epistemological continuity' is core to the quality and safety of advanced generalist care.

So we need to build epistemological continuity – a 'trial and learn' approach – into thinking about how we enable and advance medical generalist practice. We need to support patients and clinicians not only to develop and share explanations of illness, but also to agree a 'trial and learn' plan – what they expect the planned management options to achieve. Both parties put the 'trial' plan into action; either or both can be involved in the 'learning' element. Sometimes, we may invite the patient to take sole responsibility for the learning. I might suggest to Elsie and her carers that, following changes to her medication, we hope she will become more active and engaged. We certainly don't expect her mood and engagement to get worse. If they see Elsie stay well and improve, no further input or action is needed from me as the generalist clinician (at this time anyway). But if she declines again, starts becoming withdrawn again, then I will need to re-visit, explore again and re-interpret (or explain) what is happening – perhaps reconsidering the issue of depressed mood.

The generalist approach may involve Elsie receiving off protocol, or even 'beyond protocol' care. Others reviewing this care, if not involved in the inductive process, may be worried about apparent poor care and seek to change the prescribing decisions. In an ideal world, we would make decisions about a patient like Elsie in active consultation with all clinicians potentially involved in her care. In reality, that clinical team is diverse and changing. So instead it is important that we record the management plan, and justification for it, in a shared record space for Elsie. I will return to this point in Chapter 5 when I discuss the TAILOR project. Shared records can also help with epistemological continuity through expanding the team potentially involved in the trial and learn approach. Epistemological continuity, and the capacity to review and revise explanations and plans for care, is currently more easily managed in the primary care setting (in the UK at least) where follow-up may be easier to arrange. Secondary care clinicians may be hesitant about making changes to care that they can't easily follow-up and review. Improvement in shared records and communication across the extended team may help to enhance the generalist model into secondary care settings as well.

Shifting from specialist to generalist: The impact of the 4Es

In Elsie's case, I have described shifting our clinical focus from what has been described as the 'command and control' of disease-states (her blood pressure) to supporting health for daily living. This is achieved through the use of advanced generalist skills to create tailored explanations of illness and healthcare need. As I will describe in the chapters that follow, it has the potential to address some of the significant healthcare system challenges that I described in Chapter 1. I will present case studies that demonstrate how tailored whole person care can help us address the growing iatrogenic challenge of the burden of healthcare. I will show how it can re-energise healthcare clinicians demotivated by an overly bureaucratic healthcare system, allowing them to re-engage with the values and principles that brought them into medicine. I will describe how this approach underpins the development of individual and community health-related capacity for everyday living. I therefore propose a new model of advanced generalist care that strengthens the practice and delivery of primary healthcare – the system of care shown to which we know best delivers efficient, effective and equitable healthcare (Kringos et al. 2013) (Figure 2.5).

If we are to reap the benefits of strengthened generalist healthcare, we will need to make a number of changes to the way we practice. To enhance generalist Epistemology, we will need to embed the Wise framework in recognised descriptions of best practice (and best evidence for practice). For generalist exploration, we will need to augment deductive statistical testing with the actions of data discovery and integration. To strengthen generalist explanation, we will need to shift the focus from looking just for a 'correct diagnosis' to a 'tailored explanation'. For generalist evaluation, we need to replace the transactional measures of quality (pass or fail) to measures which assess capacity for and quality of learning. I shall return to a consideration of the implications for changes

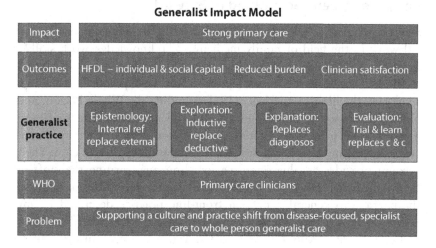

Figure 2.5   Impact model of advanced generalist practice.

in training, practice and policy that all of this brings in the chapters that follow. But before I do, let me take a brief step back to evaluate the ideas I have presented so far.

2.6 ADVANCED GENERALISM: EMPEROR'S NEW CLOTHES OR TRULY DIFFERENT?

It has taken me 2 years to write this book. In that time, many people have been calling for a culture shift in clinical practice: to improve patient-centred care and reduce the burden of care on patients. In that time, I have re-visited some of the established writing on generalist practice – the work of Stange, Gunn, and Howe as well as Stewart and McWhinney's account of the person-centred method. I explored Health Education England's plans to establish Schools of Generalism.

As I read each contribution, my question was the same: Does my account of Medical Generalism, Now! offer anything new, anything different to the accounts that have done before? Is my account of the knowledge work of generalist practice describing something new, something different? Or is it just the Emperor's new clothes – an interesting academic alternative story – but one that doesn't offer us anything new? You perhaps won't be surprised to hear that I conclude that these previous accounts don't champion knowledge work in the way needed to address modern challenges. I'll try and explain that conclusion by considering a couple of examples.

The person-centred method of Stewart

Stewart et al.'s (2003) text on patient-centred medicine is a seminal work in the field of family medicine. The knowledge work skills I describe in this book are implicit in their writing on the person-centred method. They describe six components for best practice, including: Exploring the illness experience, Understanding the Whole Person, and Finding Common Ground. Stewart and colleagues use case studies to illustrate these principles in action, and to describe the impact on person-centred care, and the therapeutic value of relationship based care. Their account provides a value reference for clinicians learning the craft of family medicine. However, it doesn't adequately recognise, or address, the barriers to generalist care in front-line practice described by my research. Stewart and colleagues' method has shaped the teaching of GPs and consultation skills for many years. Yet, it has been insufficient to challenge the guideline-dominance of current practice models in clinical reasoning. It doesn't provide a clear account of the 'permission to move beyond protocol-based care' needed to support a shift in professional skills, confidence and practice. I therefore suggest that the 4Es approach complements, and extends, Stewart and colleagues' account to address the gaps highlighted.

Shared decision making

My second consideration asks if the generalist approach I describe here is simply the same thing as the concept of shared decision making (SDM).

'No decision about me, without me' was a government catch phrase promoting person-centred care first seen in the NHS more than 10 years ago. Government, policy makers and professional bodies have long recognised a principle of best practice which involves actively engaging patients in making shared decisions about their healthcare – whether specialist or generalist. So what is the difference between shared decision making and whole person advanced generalist practice?

Once again, the difference is revealed in the epistemological approaches adopted by the two ways of working. SDM is grounded in a hypothetico-deductive reasoning approach. Specialist reasoning is used to assess the statistical probability that an individual has a disease or would benefit from a treatment. SDM is then used to decide on the personal significance of that statistical probability.

Consider the example of a person identified as having essential hypertension. Their QRisk score is calculated to describe a risk of having a heart attack or stroke in the next 20 years of – let's say – 10%. Does that warrant medical treatment? Meta-synthesis of clinical trials will tell us the probability that medical intervention would reduce this individual's risk. SDM tools help us share that information in an accessible form with patients so they can share in the medical practice of deciding if treatment is needed. There are potentially some generalist elements in this interpretation of value. However, current SDM practice doesn't change the process we use to decide if we should medicalise (diagnose) an individual with a condition or risk factor. I'll return to this point again when I consider Heath's Gatekeeper model of generalist practice in Chapter 3.

So my account not only resonates with but also extends the existing writing on generalist practice. Perhaps the key reason for Medical Generalism, Now! and its focus on knowledge work, is the recognition that existing writings have been insufficient to challenge the dominance of the disease-focused models of healthcare now recognised to be contributing to so many of the problems facing modern healthcare systems.

2.7 KNOWLEDGE WORK: THE MISSING PIECE IN PERSON-CENTRED HEALTHCARE REDESIGN

In this chapter, I discussed a shift in clinical reasoning which moves us from assessing a patient's diagnostic status to understanding their health and illness in context. I have described the scientific underpinnings of this work – the methods that enable me to confidently generate and learn from new, tailored knowledge-in-context. I have described a third model of clinical reasoning – inductive reasoning – with the Wise framework to support analysis of trustworthiness. All of which enables us to use, but also move beyond, scientific evidence to deliver healthcare tailored to the needs of our patients and communities.

But research, including my own, demonstrates that this work is being undermined and lost in modern healthcare. We have failed to design this work into the way we train healthcare professionals, run healthcare practices and set policy through healthcare strategy.

Our current health systems face huge challenges in meeting the demands upon them. Our current strategies look to find ways to make our health systems work faster and more efficiently to meet the demand – improving how clinicians use data to make disease-focused diagnoses, how patients adhere to the treatment models offered and how the health system collects the data to monitor and maintain the service.

Yet, as we get better at delivering 'the same' care at greater speed and volume, we are generating a new iatrogenic problem – that of treatment burden. Being able to deliver more disease-focused care, at scale and speed, is adding to the emerging new problem of modern healthcare – that of treatment burden and iatrogenic harm. Just as Illich predicted it would, the healthcare intended to make things better is actually becoming part of the problem.

If we want to reverse this trend and restore strong person-centred primary care, we need to tackle the missing piece in primary care redesign – the knowledge work of expert generalist practice. In the next chapters, I will consider how we can do just that.

REFERENCES

Bliss M. (1999). William Osler: A Life in Medicine. Oxford, England: Oxford University Press.

Coady D, Chase J (Eds). (2019). The Routledge Handbook of Applied Epistemology. Oxon: Routledge.

Croskerry P. (2009). A universal model of diagnostic reasoning. American Medicine, 84, pp. 1022–1028.

Donner-Banzhoff H, Hertwig R. (2014). Inductive foraging: Improving the diagnostic yield of primary care consultations. European Journal of General Practice, 20, pp. 69–73.

Gabbay J, le May A. (2011). Practice-based evidence for healthcare. Clinical Mindlines. Oxon: Routledge.

Gabbay J, le May A. (2023). Knowledge Transformation in Health and Social Care. Oxon: Routledge.

Henegan C et al. (2009). Diagnostic strategies used in primary care. BMJ, 338, p. b946.

Kings Fund. (2013). Polypharmacy and Medicines Optimisation. London: Kings Fund.

Kringos D et al. (2013). The strength of primary care in Europe: An international comparative study. British Journal of General Practice, 63, pp. e742–750.

Kvale S. (1996). Interview Views: An Introduction to Qualitative Research Interviewing. Thousand Oaks, CA: Sage Publications.

Kvale S, Brinkmann S. (2008). Interviews: Learning the Craft of Qualitative Research Interviewing. Thousand Oaks, CA: SAGE Publications.

May CR et al. (2015). Normalisation Process Theory. https://normalization-process-theory.northumbria.ac.uk/

Müskens JLJM, Kool RB, van Dulmen SA, Westert GP. (2022). Overuse of diagnostic testing in healthcare: a systematic review. BMJ Quality & Safety, 31, pp. 54–63.

NICE. (2018). Guideline NG84. www.nice.org.uk/guidance/ng84/chapter/Summary-of-the-evidence

Nonaka I, Takeuchi H. (1995) The Knowledge Creating Company. New York: Oxford University Press.

Reeve J. (2010). Interpretive medicine: Supporting generalism in a changing primary care world. Occasional Paper Series Royal College of General Practitioners, 88, pp. 1–20.

Sackett DL et al. (1991). Clinical Epidemiology: A Basic Science for Clinical Medicine. Lippincott Williams & Wilkins.

Sackett DL et al. (1996). Evidence-based medicine: what it is, and what it isn't. BMJ, 321, p. 71. https://www.bmj.com/content/312/7023/71.full

Scambler G. (2018). Sociology as Applied to Health and Medicine. London: Palgrave.

Seale C, Pattison S. (2001). Medical Knowledge: Doubt and Uncertainty (2nd edition). Buckinghamshire: Open University Press.

Skultans V. (2003). From damaged nerves to masked depression: Inevitability and hope in Latvian psychiatric narratives. Social Science & Medicine, 56, pp. 2421–2431.

Stewart M et al. (2003). Patient-Centered Medicine, Transforming the Clinical Method (2nd edition). Radcliffe Medical Press.

Watson JC. (n.d.) Epistemic Justification. Internet Encyclopaedia of Philosophy. https://iep.utm.edu/epi-just/

Wenzel RP. (2017). Medical education in an era of alternative facts. New England Journal of Medicine, 377, pp. 607–609.

CHAPTER 3

Wise people: Delivering the knowledge work of expert generalist practice

....

In my first two chapters, I outlined the principles of advanced generalist practice – tailored healthcare grounded in the distinct knowledge work of whole person healthcare, supporting health for daily living for individuals and communities. In the next three chapters, I will focus on what that looks like on the ground, in daily practice. Using practical examples of generalist care in action from my own work and colleagues, I will highlight the distinct knowledge work contribution in each. From there, I will consider how these examples challenge and potentially re-shape current healthcare practice and policy.

In the first of these three chapters, I start with a look at the work that happens in the interaction between a patient and a clinician – at the level of the consultation. I will explore three examples of applied knowledge work that demonstrate a different generalist approach to consulting – the BOUNCEBACK project, Goldilocks Medicine and the Generalist Guru. This chapter will again demonstrate why the generalist physician is no jack of all trades, master of none; but rather uses an advanced form of professional practice perhaps better characterised as 'mastery within all trades'.

So let's start with the case of an innovation project we ran a few years ago to bring advanced generalist thinking into everyday practice – the BOUNCEBACK project. This work described a new tool for generalist practice – the Flipped Consultation.

DOI: 10.1201/9781003297222-3

3.1 THE FLIPPED CONSULTATION

Ten years ago, we set out to develop and test an innovative approach to generalist care within the BOUNCEBACK project. This was a local innovation project which brought together partners from general practice, a mental health charity (AiW Health) and Liverpool University. Our goal was to explore whether we could design and deliver an alternative model of care for common mental health problems seen in everyday primary care practice, using generalist, whole person principles. I'll talk more in Chapter 4 about the practice-level redesign elements of this work. Here, I want to focus on what we learnt about redesigning the way we work with individual patients – how we rethink the consultation.

Pendleton described the consultation as 'the central act of medicine'. General practice has long recognised the person-centred consultation as its core tool. Consultation skills are integral to the identity of the discipline of general practice. The consultation is a meeting between (at least) two parties – the patient and the clinician. (Swinglehurst [2019] also recognises a third party – the computer). Students of general practice are taught consultation models that are designed to establish and support good communication between these parties. These models are grounded in an understanding of the biopsychosocial model of clinical practice. I'm going to start by taking a closer look at that approach, before considering how and why BOUNCEBACK worked differently.

The biopsychosocial model of medicine was first described in 1977 by George Engel – an internist and psychiatrist working in America. An internist is a doctor who manages 'internal organ systems', without specialising in one system; and is usually based in a hospital. So an internist is a generalist physician – potentially able to manage many different problems and sharing professional roles with the GP.

Engel described that to understand human illness, we had to look at more than the biomedical (pathological) elements (Engel 1977). Biomedicine can describe what has gone wrong in a body system – the deviation from physiological, anatomical and biochemical norm that defines a disease state. This can give us some insight into what has happened (e.g., an artery has blocked causing ischaemia of the heart) and what symptoms we might expect the patient to experience (chest pain, shortness of breath). But to truly understand what has happened, we need also to consider the psychological (mood, personality, behaviours) and social (cultural, familial, socio-economic) elements that have contributed to the pathological processes happening, the symptoms experienced and the resources available to manage the illness related disruption. The biopsychosocial model recognises that different individual patients may have very different symptoms and experiences from the same underlying pathological process, and also different responses to management. In its original form, the biopsychosocial model requires us to tailor both diagnostic and management processes to the individual in front of us.

Consultation models grounded in the biopsychosocial model are therefore intended to collect data on each element of the biological, psychological and social. For example, does this person have symptoms suggestive of a pathological process (history of the complaint and past history); how are daily activities and behaviours affected and contributing to this; and what lifestyle and social context factors might be contributing to the problem and how we manage it? In practice, the biopsychosocial model is more commonly used to shape management than diagnosis. Consultation models typically start with a biomedical exploration of the current problem and previous medical history. Later on, we may explore the behavioural and social factors that both contribute to the illness experience (for example, smoking status) and how the individual responds to their illness (for example, their social support network). Driven by the hypothetico-deductive approach, consultations essentially look to assess a biomedical explanation for the illness, and then consider the wider factors that may need to be addressed in its management.

For example, consider the (again, fictitious) case of Anna. She is a young woman in her twenties who presents feeling tired all the time with a productive cough and shortness of breath. Her 'bio' history suggests she has a lower respiratory tract infection. The 'psychosocial' elements identify that she is a smoker and a single mum living in a damp flat on the 12th floor of a high-rise block. Her smoking is identified as a risk factor for her chest infection and she is referred to a smoking cessation service. But although we have used a biopsychosocial approach in this consultation, we have not necessarily explored the broader issues about why Anna smokes (Oakley 1989), or indeed why she is feeling tired all the time. We have used a person-centred approach to shape our management of the problem, but we haven't used a generalist approach to diagnosis.

BOUNCEBACK set out to introduce a whole-person-centred approach to both the diagnosis and management of mild to moderate distress in people presenting to primary care services. To do this, it aimed to reverse the traditional biopsychosocial approach and instead work from the social to the psychological before considering the biomedical. In

Chapter 4, I'll describe the changes we needed to make at the practice level to enable this work to happen. Here, I want to focus on the work we did to change the interaction between patient and clinician. To introduce whole person mental healthcare in practice, we developed a new approach to consulting – what we described as the Flipped Consultation model. Embedded within this was the Exhaustion Cycle. These two tools enabled us to introduce an advanced generalist clinical model into everyday primary care practice. So let me describe what we did.

At the time we were running the BOUNCEBACK project, NICE guidelines were encouraging clinicians to use a stepped care approach to assessing and managing mild-moderate depression in the primary care setting. When a patient presented with symptoms of low mood or distress, clinicians were encouraged to use a validated tool to assess mood such as PHQ9. If the patient met the criteria for depression, the clinician was encouraged to use their PHQ9 score to guide the treatment approach using stepped care. Essentially mild depression (low scores) could be managed with psychoeducation and support. For people with moderate scores, clinicians were encouraged to consider referral for cognitive behavioural therapy. High scores should prompt consideration of the use of medication, with or without psychological therapy. Secondary care, specialist input, was reserved for severe cases or people with other risk factors for poor outcomes. Primary care clinicians, trained in the biopsychosocial approach, were encouraged to explore the contextual factors that might impact an individual's capacity to use the recommended treatment approach. Effectively, we are using biopsychosocial approaches to optimise management of the biomedically defined condition.

The BOUNCEBACK team argued for an alternative approach. The primary driver for our work was recognised concerns about the unintended consequences of medicalising an illness experience of distress. Debates have raged for many decades on the over, and under, diagnosis of depression, and indeed the over, and under, use of antidepressant medication for people experiencing distress. But the BOUNCEBACK team had clinical experience from NHS and charity settings of both the potentially unintended negative impacts of medicalising distress, and of the positive effects that can be seen when using alternative approaches. So we set out to critically examine the feasibility of embedding alternative non-medicalisation approaches to assessment and management of distress into the general practice setting. If we found it was possible to do, our goal was to formally compare the impact of socio-psycho-bio approaches with biopsychosocial consultations.

I have already said the team had clinical experience of using different ways of looking at and managing mild-moderate distress. AiW was a local mental health charity with extensive experience of working with people experiencing significant distress. People presenting to AiW case workers described experiencing significant disruption to their daily lives due to the effect of distress, low mood and poor concentration. AiW staff would work with clients to understand the context in which people were living with and experiencing these problems, as well as the resources they had to support their creative capacity and the flow of daily living (ballast, sources of power and contributors to stability). Together, they would then look to find ways to strengthen the resources and lessen the load. This non-medical approach to managing distress had been successful over many years.

As we planned the BOUNCEBACK project, we also explored the research evidence that supports a demedicalisation approach to managing mild to moderate mental health. My PhD, for example, looked at the benefits and harm of medicalising distress in people living with terminal cancer. Part of that work involved interviewing patients (using a travelling approach) to explore their experiences of distress and how they dealt with it. The stories they told me almost all rejected a biomedical view that their distress was a 'disease state' (depression). Participants instead described their distress as arising from the work they were doing to juggle the many demands they faced, navigating through the choppy waters of the flow of daily living, with falling energy levels as their illness progressed and varying anchors and ballast to balance that all out (Chapter 1). Those interviews described a strong narrative of biographical flow – of maintaining daily living even in the face of significant adverse events. Disruption did happen – episodes which those affected described as periods of depression. These occurred when the demands on individuals outweighed the resources available to them. For example, one person hit their low time when exhausted by the effects of chemotherapy. For others, the imbalance arose from events in their personal life. Most people recognised a background low-level distress as part of their experience of living with, and dying from, cancer. But as one participant described to me, 'It's not depression, it's a quiet mode of deep thinking'.

The approach used by AiW is also recognised in the writing of Emmy Gut (1989) – a psychologist who talks about a concept of 'productive depression'. She described that when we are overwhelmed by factors in our daily life, we may enter a period of depressed mood as a protective response. Withdrawing from our usual everyday activities, as a result of lowering mood, can potentially be seen as a positive or productive response to adverse events. By stopping doing our usual work, this may allow us time, space and energy for the recharge and reflection needed to respond differently. This was certainly the experience of AiW case workers supporting clients who presented with feelings of being overwhelmed or exhausted. Encouraging people to take some time out from, or perhaps handing over responsibility for, some of their everyday (routine) work was often a valuable first step in helping to life their clients' mood.

Whilst I was doing my PhD, a patient came to see me in practice to tell me 'my depression is back, I need to re-start my medication'. Let's call him Frank. Frank described feeling overwhelmed, tired all the time and low in mood. He was still managing to go to work, but every day was feeling harder. He was a successful business man, happily married and had a holiday home he could 'escape' to. Yet, he was feeling low. His experience of having been here before was that he would need to take antidepressants for 6 months or so and that would sort things out.

I started a conversation with Frank on the lines of the work of maintaining biographical flow that I had explored with the participants in my PhD. Frank found this conversation gave him a completely different understanding of his illness experience and his options for managing it. We discussed his exhaustion and feeling overwhelmed. Frank reflected that the things he usually did to look after himself in the face of the usual demands of his job and everyday life (booking a holiday, for example) were no longer enough to correct the imbalance that had crept in. In terms of the ideas we discussed in Chapter 1, the anchors and power that came from his creative self were not enough to balance things. Frank had become overwhelmed and exhausted.

Our conversation explored the many factors contributing to Frank's current experience of illness. Through this, we created a new explanation of how he was feeling. Frank started to consider that there might be an alternative approach to restarting his antidepressants. He chose instead to go and reflect on our conversation with his family and friends, and to explore alternative ways of 're-balancing'. Unfortunately for me, I never got to meet with Frank again and find out more about what happened. But I do know that Frank didn't come back into the practice for management of his 'depression' (or move practices for those of you who are wondering). So he had certainly found an alternative approach, and presumably one that was at least as effective as medicalisation.

All of this fed into our BOUNCEBACK conversations about how we might redesign the way we approach people presenting with mild to moderate distress. We worked out that we wanted to turn the biopsychosocial consultation model upside down. We would start our conversations with someone presenting in distress by exploring the 'social' aspects – their work of daily living, considering if and how that contributed to an explanation of their distress. We'd then work with the patient to put things in place to help – social and psychological support – to help with the work. Only if this didn't help would we consider exploring a biomedical option for understanding and managing distress. We called this the Flipped Consultation model (Lucassen 2018).

In a Flipped Consultation, we would explore with people the work of daily living, and the resources they had (or were missing) to help with that work. We'd invite people to reflect, like Frank, on the balance, or imbalance, between demands and resources – and to think about what effect that was having on their health and wellbeing. Our goal was to use the expertise of both the health worker and the patient to explore options for doing things differently: recognising distress as a sign of the need for change, and using shared expertise to identify and implement things that could help. In practice, these conversations often revealed that people needed help with social elements such as housing, finance or work. Sometimes, there would be psychological elements that needed some behavioural activation approaches to help the person start doing things differently. The consultation would openly discuss what changes we were expecting to see as a result of the plans we made. We'd book in a plan to meet and review and evaluate the plan. Our 'safety net' was always a biomedical approach – referral to, and discussion with, a GP.

BOUNCEBACK was an innovation study. We were funded to explore if it was possible to introduce a new way of working into usual general practice – was it possible to integrate charity case workers into practice, and so change the model of care provision. The project wasn't designed as a clinical trial – to generate statistical assessment of the impact of the changes. But it did generate important case study evidence. Evaluation of the BOUNCEBACK pilot demonstrated both a beneficial impact on a patient's capacity for daily living and self-management and also improved professional satisfaction. We have since used the BOUNCEBACK approach to develop professional education resources for clinicians including the Exhaustion Cycle – see Box 3.1. Professional reflection and case studies have demonstrated positive impact for patients and clinicians alike.

BOX 3.1 DESCRIBING THE EXHAUSTION CYCLE

The Exhaustion Cycle recognises socio-psycho-bio explanations for the mild-moderate distress commonly presented to primary care as anxiety or depressed mood (Figure 3.1). It focuses on an individual's work of daily living and the creative capacity of individuals to manage that work. The model recognises that if the work to do starts to consistently exceed our capacity to deliver, the result is an uneven seesaw and the potential for an 'exhaustion crash'.

Starting at the top of the cycle, we recognise that human beings are 'wired up' to maintain homeostasis – to keep things in balance. We can think about our daily work in terms of the balance (or imbalance) between the work we do, and the energy we have to do it. Things that 'drain' our energy include everyday activities like keeping a roof over our head, food on the table; but also looking after ourselves and our families and friends. We use up energy going to work, but also on activities

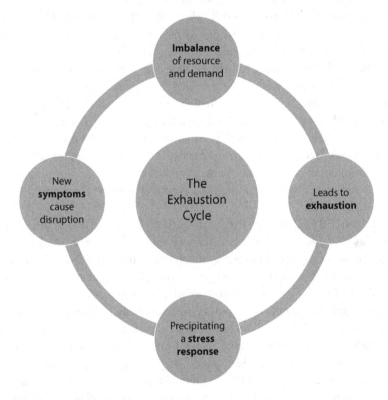

Figure 3.1   The Exhaustion Cycle.

that we enjoy. Many of these activities also appear on the 'balance' side of our see saw. Food on the table, time with our families, hobbies and activities all give us energy back too. (My discussion of creative capacity and Maslow's hierarchy explores all of this too.)

If the resources and demands get out of balance, we experience a net 'drain' on our energy levels. It's like having a leaky bucket – even if we try and top up its never enough to get us back to a healthy 'energy level'.

The result is that we become exhausted – chronically tired. But if we have to keep going, even just with the everyday things, then we start to rely on a 'spare battery' – the stress hormones that (appear to) keep us going.

Adrenaline bursts give us the energy to do things, but also cause a whole host of new symptoms for us to deal with: fogginess, exaggerated pain responses, poor sleep, a feeling of being tired all the time. These symptoms, and the worry they cause us, act as a further drain on our 'out-of-balance' seesaw. And so we spiral around in a cycle of exhaustion.

We can use this cycle to explore a person's experience of distress, also helping them to recognise these elements and so make sense of what is happening. The cycle also gives us four additional points of intervention: implementing strategies to 'recharge the batteries' of a leaky bucket (if you'll forgive the mixed meta-phors!); considering the use of beta-blockers to amend the adrenaline response; helping the individual recognise the additional symptoms they are experiencing as 'trigger points' – a sign they need to stop, do something different; and cognitive behavioural therapy to help work on the (often ingrained) behaviours contributing to out of balance seesaw.

The Flipped Consultation approach used the Exhaustion Cycle to explore, explain and manage distress as a starting point; only 'escalating' to biomedical considerations if distress persisted. A Flipped Consultation focuses on whole per-son management of an experience of distress, mobilising the resources of the individual and their community as first line. I have written more on this approach in my chapter on the Creative Self (Reeve 2019).

The BOUNCEBACK project also focused on the wider practice arrangements that needed to change to support this approach. I'll dis-cuss that more in Chapter 4. But the consultation element described here illustrates the use of the 4Es in practice. The Flipped Consultation is grounded in the knowledge work of advanced generalist practice.

The knowledge work of the flipped consultation

Essentially, the Flipped Consultation and Exhaustion Cycle are tools supporting the knowledge work of daily generalist practice – the work needed to explore, explain and evaluate implementation of a tailored understanding of illness disrupting everyday life. The tools give the whole person clinician a framework by which to explore and explain the experience of health-related disruption to daily living, considering the range of factors that may be contributing to distress. In Frank's case, he recognised being overwhelmed and exhausted by all the plates he was juggling and exhausted. His exhaustion lowered his mood. He was unable to take time out, and so adrenaline was keeping him going, but adding to his anxiety.

The Flipped Consultation approach offered a way to involve Frank in the knowledge work of making sense of his illness, in the work of whole person care. By helping Frank explore the range of factors impacting on his whole person health and developing explanations (through the Exhaustion Cycle) of how life-work was contributing to his illness experience, Frank became part of the creative team managing his depressed mood. The knowledge work became part of the therapeutic process. Similar patients I have worked with since have described how this account has helped them to shift their interpretation of the cause of her illness. They no longer see their mood problems as a biochemical problem in their brain that can only be managed with medication, but instead an issue of an imbalance which they can be part of managing, with the support of others.

The Flipped Consultation is a model which is grounded in the principles I described in Chapter 1. Including health for daily living; recognising healthcare as only one small component of health; and empowering the creative capacity of the self in order to understand and manage distress. It is a model which is valued by patients – who welcome the explanation, the opportunity to enhance their own creative capacity and to develop their ability to manage similar future problems. It is also a model appreciated by clinicians – including for the situations where they seek to support patients who are not 'responding' (gaining benefit) from antidepressants. The Flipped Consultation gives an alternative approach to exploring these patients' illness than having to repeatedly cycle round new antidepressants. Given that current healthcare practice is querying the overuse of antidepressant medication, and the overmedicalisation of distress, the Flipped Consultation model describes and approach that is informed by evidence, relies on knowledge work to explore, explain and evaluate distress, and is consistent with a goal to de-medicalise and de-escalate iatrogenesis.

But it is a model which needs a rethink of the practice set up and consultation approaches needed to deliver. It needs time (it is not a 10-minute consultation), continuity between practitioner and patient to explore and learn from the narrative created and shared record of the management approach across wider teams to ensure consistency of approach. The Flipped Consultation is a tool for Wise People (practitioners with advanced knowledge work skills for generalist practice) but it also demonstrates that delivery will need Wise Places to support its use in practice. I will return to this point in Chapter 4.

3.2 GOLDILOCKS MEDICINE

My second case study also looked at both patient and practice-level changes needed to support the knowledge work of whole person practice. This time, it focuses on 'physical' rather than 'mental' health aspects (although from a whole person perspective, the division is artificial). I am going to take a look at one of the biggest challenges facing modern healthcare – the burden(s) of multimorbidity and chronic illness.

When the UK established the core elements of its primary care/ general practice service in 1948, healthcare was mainly dealing with acute illness – infections, trauma – and events – pregnancy, death. (For GPs, this included more 'acute' mental health issues – the distress of bereavement and loss.) But the key issue was that the health service was designed to treat and manage shorter-term problems.

Since then, the epidemiology of healthcare need has changed beyond recognition. Two features stand out: the shift from acute to chronic illness, and from single to multiple, complex illness. A growing proportion of the population live their lives with a chronic health problem – something that can't be cured, but instead requires ongoing management. As more people live with long-term illness, so we also see growing numbers living with more than one condition – a phenomenon described as multimorbidity. Barnett et al's (2012) groundbreaking paper in the *Lancet* offered a powerful visual representation of a growing 'tsunami' of multimorbidity associated with aging populations living with a growing burden of chronic illnesses. People have also described a new concept of 'frailty' – recognising that aging individuals and populations have altered biopsychosocial capacity to deal with illness. In the context of generalist medicine, recognising health as a resource for daily living, frailty can be understood as a reduced capacity to accommodate health- and illness-related challenges to daily life. In addition 20% of consultations in general practice in England are for what have been described as Medically Unexplained Symptoms or Persistent Physical Symptoms (Rosendal et al. 2017). An estimated 3–10% of adult patients registered with general practice have long-term medically explained symptoms. In general practice, 3–10% of adult patients have long-term medically unexplained symptoms. These are patients living with, and managing the work of, chronic health problems but without a clear diagnosis to guide them.

All this means that modern healthcare systems, including primary care, are dealing with growing numbers of people living with the burden of persistent health problems – some biomedically defined, but many not so. Yet, patients are also living with the burden of healthcare for those conditions. Our knowledge of what we can do to manage disease continues to grow rapidly as illustrated, for example, by the volume of new published evidence for practice. Guidelines describe many 'options' for care of each condition they address. For the individual who lives with multiple conditions, the list of 'options' becomes potentially overwhelming. I explored this in Chapter 1 when I introduced Hughes et al.'s (2013) work on the burden of guidelines care for frail elders. This highlighted how the burden of healthcare on daily living can quickly start to outweigh the burden of living with illness – the very thing it was intended to help (see May et al. 2009; Tran et al. 2012 in Chapter 1). Anyone reading this book who is either a practising clinician, or a patient or carer of someone living with long-term illness, will have personal experience of the burden placed on patients by modern healthcare.

Our knowledge of what we *can* do for the management of disease continues to grow rapidly. However, our mechanisms for dealing with the related question – what *should* we do – are far less developed. Understanding how we get things *just right* for an individual is the goal of a concept I have described as Goldilocks Medicine. This concept involves us in balancing a number of considerations, such as asking what could we do to manage conditions medically, and what would be the implications for the individual's work of daily living including their creative capacity (positive and negative). What alternative approaches might we consider and what might be the implications of not managing the problem medically. All of this involves clinician and patient in the generation of a tailored explanation of illness and its management.

A number of years ago, I was involved in a project that used the Goldilocks approach to try and improve the care we were offering to frail older people living at home with multiple long-term conditions. This was the Complex Needs project. The project, again, involved making changes in how we organised practice care to support these patients. I'll discuss all that further in Chapter 4. Here, I want to focus on what we learnt from that work about the consultation process – working with individual patients. The Complex Needs work demonstrates the 4Es in action.

Epistemology: The framework for the project

In the Complex Needs project, we aimed to change how we supported vulnerable housebound patients living with complex illness – multiple long-term conditions. Our goal was to move away from managing chronic disease (and the occasional acute exacerbations) to developing and delivering care that optimised health for daily living. Within the Complex Needs project, Goldilocks care – best practice – involved optimising the input and role of primary medical care in supporting the daily living of individuals and their creative capacity. If we were to tailor care, we needed to be able to develop a tailored understanding of the options for care. The team involved in this work recognised we needed the inductive approach Type I discussed in Chapter 2 – an epistemology for whole person healthcare. Our first step was to give ourselves permission to adopt this alternative approach and to potentially work outside of guidelines.

Exploration for sense making

Next comes the practice of exploration. All of the patients in the Complex Needs project were housebound. Exploration of their illness experience meant visiting them at home. This element of the work meant that in a typical day, each Goldilocks clinician might see just eight patients. There are, of course, practical implications of this and I will return to this point. But the rationale behind requiring a GP home visit for a whole person assessment was a commitment to the second E of advanced generalist practice – that of Exploration.

For most of the duration of this project, there were two GPs involved in delivering the work. Before we went to visit a patient on our Complex Needs list, we undertook a comprehensive review and update of the individual's clinical notes. Clinical problem lists on practice systems were updated to only include active problems potentially impacting on daily living; to include a summary of the diagnosis, development and prognosis for each condition; and to update on which clinical team members (including hospital specialists) were still involved. Medication lists were similarly updated to understand why medicines had been started, intended impact (and whether any record of that had been achieved) and intended review/stop date. Inevitably, this flagged many gaps in the picture and many questions to explore with patients. There was some opportunity to explore guidelines, evidence and specialist (consultant)-level perspectives on any or all of these issues.

Non-acute planned home visits were arranged for a conversation typically lasting 45–60 minutes which followed the 'travelling' conversation model I introduced in Chapter 2. My colleague and I used Flipped Consultation-type approaches to understand, first, the individual in context – their health for daily living, and their perception of what might help and what didn't. We could then explore the biomedical issues raised by our notes review, including the questions identified. In many cases, we also spoke with carers and family who added additional information into our exploratory pot.

Once again, let me try and illustrate all this with a case study – a fictional patient, but based on a number of people I saw during the project. Farzi was a 70-year-old man. His notes review revealed that he lived alone, having lost his wife in the last couple of years. He had diagnoses of type 2 diabetes mellitus, hypertension, arthritis and prostatism and was currently taking 10 medicines a day. Most of the questions arising from his notes review related to understanding his personal experience of living with these conditions and the impact and value of his extensive medication list.

When I arrived to see Farzi, he told me he had been feeling tired all the time for many weeks and months. Using a Flipped Consultation approach, we together identified a number of factors that were contributing to him feeling overwhelmed. There is always a risk that we focus on one element in a consultation – maybe his sugar being too high, or his loneliness since losing his wife. By looking at all the data I had – medical, personal and professional – I could start to work with Farzi on our next stage.

Explanation for action

The Complex Needs project gave us a previously unheard of space for exploration but also the time to start to construct an explanation with our patients. Before this project, patients on the Complex Needs register had received an annual review assessing guideline described quality of care for each of their defined conditions. Now we were able to take a step back and consider with our patients: What are we trying to achieve? We could construct an explanation of everyday health and illness that drew on, but wasn't dictated by, existing diagnoses and sometimes new ones. That process allowed us to formulate a plan to support health for daily living: one that set clear, and sometimes new, goals for actions.

Often, this involved us in deprescribing – stopping medicines that were no longer helpful in the new tailored understanding and management plan. For some people, this also meant de-diagnosing: removing diagnoses from active problem lists and from the focus of current care planning. Our Goldilocks consultations allowed us to (critically) create a new explanation for action.

Returning to Farzi, he told us he was feeling tired all the time. His annual bloods showed that his diabetic control was suboptimal. It would be tempting to start with an assumption that his diabetes is causing the tiredness and so focus on adjusting his medication. But as Donner-Banzhoff described, this approach may shut down our considerations too soon. We might miss other elements contributing to how Farzi is feeling such as his ongoing sadness at losing his wife. In a Goldilocks approach, our goal is to explore and negotiate with Farzi a way of making sense of how he is feeling and so consider what options may be available. Our tailored explanation of his illness in context helps create an understanding of what we can do, or at least try, and also what we might expect to happen as a result. In Farzi's case, we recognise that his diabetes isn't optimally controlled, but it's also not much different to a year ago. We decide we need to consider other things too, and so agree to put Farzi in touch with the social prescribing link worker to offer him some bereavement support. We agree that we will check in with him in 3 months' time to see how he is getting on. If his sadness if lifting but his tiredness remains, we may want to consider other approaches. To some extent, this is similar to the safety netting described in consultation models such as the Inner Consultation model (Neighbour 2005) – putting a plan in place in case we have made the wrong decision. But in this case, we are going further. There is no 'right and wrong' answer here. Instead, there is an ongoing opportunity to explore and amend our explanation of illness. A 'trial and learn' approach – undertaken thoughtfully and critically – is an important part of best practice in the knowledge work of advanced generalist care.

Evaluation: Review and revise

The trial and learn approach is part of the fourth E – Evaluation. We can follow-up, review, revise and learn from inductive-based care for individual patients as in Farzi's case. We can also evaluate the care we offer to a group of patients – such as all of those involved in the Complex Needs project.

Care for all of the patients in our Complex Needs project involved an evaluation of what we had learned from our interaction(s). However, the way this evaluation worked varied between different people. Usual care for the patients in this project involved an annual chronic disease review, along with urgent visits when needed for acute illness. For a proportion of the patients we saw in this work, the extended consultation (exploration and explanation) work revealed that the care we offered was – medically speaking – no different to the usual care I have just described. We noticed that a proportion of our patients had their healthcare needs met by 'usual' chronic disease management care. Sometimes, we identified problems patients were experiencing but which fell outside of the remit of primary care and general practice. In these cases, we helped people contact community support, social support but their medical management didn't need much change. In both these scenarios, the 'evaluation' work can be passed to the patient. We have agreed what we expect to happen with the medical care agreed to date. If this is the case, we can see you again at your annual review. But if things don't go as expected, get in touch and we will review together.

However, in a majority of cases (around 70% of the patients on our Complex Needs register), a Goldilocks care approach led to clinically significant changes in their care planning and so the need for ongoing review (a trial and learn approach). These cases recognised that continuity of care was vital to the quality and robustness of the knowledge work of Goldilocks Medicine and advanced generalist practice. However, this was not continuity to support relationship-based care, but what I sometimes describe as epistemological continuity – supporting ongoing exploration, explanation and evaluation of care. As I will return to in Chapter 5 when I discuss the TAILOR project, epistemological continuity does not rely on relationship between two individuals, but rather a continuity of approach between patient and service. Continuity matters, but not necessarily in the ways we have previously described it. We need to factor this into the redesign of primary care services

Beyond the 4Es: Triage and sharing

Our experience of working differently with patients with complex needs flagged two additional factors that we need to consider in the redesign of primary for advanced generalist care. Firstly, we recognised that not all 'complex patients' are complex in the same way. Some people needed more input than others, and different people benefited from different types of input. We realised we needed to think about how we triage people with complex healthcare needs into different parts of our service.

Triage is a hot topic in today's UK general practice, although the concept is nothing new. Triage refers to how we assess the urgency and nature of an individual's need for healthcare – deciding who do they need to see and when. Traditionally in UK general practice, this role has largely been done by receptionists working with patients. A wealth of experience and expertise helps reception staff to assess the urgency of need and allocate patients to the appropriate service. As demand for our service has arisen, and indeed exceeded the capacity for supply, many general practice organisations are moving to use of digital technology to help with this assessment process. Patients complete online survey tools which explore why they are seeking help. Clinicians then review that data and triage patients on the basis of the patient reported needs and concerns. There is a long-term goal within digital healthcare to develop triage algorithms that can replace the clinician element of this process. Digital systems seek also to potentially present the clinician who then sees the patient with a provisional diagnosis based on the data collected at the time of booking the appointment. The reasoning behind such digital triage systems is currently deductive – hypothesis testing, reflecting the specialist (disease/condition) focused design of modern healthcare.

In the Complex Needs project, we recognised that whole person assessment involves an additional element in this assessment, or triage, process. The work involves not just assessing what disease processes may be present (and how urgent are they), but also does this individual need whole person (inductive), or condition-specific (deductive) care, or even both. A GP has skills in both specialist and advanced generalist care, whilst other healthcare professionals in the growing primary care team have different skill sets. We need to get better at identifying which type of care patients need – based on their candidacy or capacity to benefit from different types of care – so that we can better allocate patient need to professional group.

Traditionally, triage processes focus on risk assessment – asking does this individual have a problem needing immediate biomedical management. The patient with crushing chest pain, symptoms of sepsis or acute neurological signs doesn't need a whole person assessment but signposting urgently to acute specialist care. For others, the risk may not be immediate, but with a clear indication of the need for specialist care. For example, the person with Parkinson's disease who needs their medication adjusted to prevent prolonged episodes of 'freezing' first needs condition-specific (specialist) input, with potential for other roles to follow. But that same individual presenting feeling 'tired all the time' potentially needs a whole person assessment to explore the extent of the problem, to develop a tailored explanation and implement and evaluate an approach to dealing with their experienced disruption to daily living.

Currently, once we have filtered out the urgent, acute cases, all others go through as 'undifferentiated need' to a range of primary care health professions. At this stage, clinician and patient undertake an additional process of assessing candidacy. Etz et al. (2021) describe this as the prioritisation role for the generalist – a process of 'sorting, ranking and negotiating what is most important'. They describe this as 'the most under-recognised and unique function of primary care within the healthcare enterprise'. One aspect of this work is the inductive foraging introduced in Chapter 2. Throughout this exploration process, the advanced generalist practitioner is undertaking a rapid critical evaluation and judgement of the data they are collecting to understand what approach of care is needed. This is a 'generalist triage' process. So how do we do that?

Reflecting on my own practice, as well as the findings from multiple research studies, I recognise a number of techniques that I use in my exploration of a patient's first contact with me. The first relates to frequency of contact with healthcare. As I am writing this chapter, UK general practice is dealing with an overwhelming demand for care – with around 33 million consultations delivered every month. In 2019, people consulted with their GP on average four times a year. In 2022, it was six to seven times a year; and in my day-to-day practice, I commonly see people who have presented five to six times in the last month. The reasons for these multiple presentations are complex. Some relate to patient, and societal factors; many relate to problems with the way we are running health services. But in my daily practice, if I see anyone who has had more than one or two consultations in the last couple of months with us then my 'generalist radar' is alerted. Repeated contact with healthcare suggests we are not adequately explaining and addressing health concerns, and flags up the need for a new exploratory approach. I will usually try to arrange a face-to-face generalist review with these patients.

A quick look at someone's medical history will also give me some pointers. Anyone with multiple long-term conditions, or who is on multiple long-term medicines, will already be potentially on my list for a generalist review to assess, at a minimum, the workload they are living with. Then there is the presenting problem – described either to a receptionist, or in an online appointment request form. As I have described, urgent triage processes should have filtered out high-risk issues. Of the people remaining, some will have biomedical needs – often clearly stated by the patient when they are seeking an appointment (for example, 'I have an ingrowing toe nail and it's not clearing'). But many patients will express more diffuse illness experience – persistent symptoms, unexplained symptoms or uncertainty about managing ongoing conditions. Patients seeking help for vague, poorly defined or multiple symptoms trigger my generalist radar and allocation to a generalist assessment, usually face to face to optimise a 'travelling' over a 'mining' conversation.

Linked to the presenting problem is the patient's 'opening pitch' when they first speak with a clinician. The generalist consultation is a conversation, and a negotiation, between experts. Patients come with expert knowledge of their work of daily living and the impact of their illness. Increasingly, they also bring knowledge about their illness that they have gained from social networks and social media. In my 20+ years of GP practice, this has always been part of general practice (e.g., 'my mum said I should come and see you'). The difference now is that patients may come with already formed ideas about 'diagnoses' that they have gained from the internet or even private sector assessments. The prioritising role of the generalist clinician described by Etz et al. has become even more complex. They may be required first to understand, untangle and possibly dismantle, explanations that have been previously formed so that the generalist clinician and patient can start to build a new robust, whole person account. The boundaries between triage, assessment and diagnosis or the formation of explanation become ever more complex.

These reflections also resonate with the second 'added extra' of generalist care that we observed within the Complex Needs work: namely the importance of shared working across a team. Patients being seen by the Complex Needs team were often also being supported by other members of wider primary and secondary care teams. Goldilocks care plans recorded in the general practice notes were not always accessible to these wider team members. On a couple of occasions, this led to misunderstandings about the reasoning and intentions behind clinical decision making – creating confusion for the clinician and patient alike. Just as we had noted in the BOUNCEBACK work, the important of communication and sharing tailored explanations and management plans clearly across diverse teams was vital. Traditional record keeping approaches were usually not enough to manage this. One simple change we introduced was to 'flag' patients being managed under the Complex Needs approach within their recorded Clinical Problem list – the summary record seen when first accessing a patient's notes – by adding a clinical code and brief explanation. Shared record keeping was a challenge we didn't solve during the Complex Needs work, but would certainly need to be addressed in any future delivery of care.

Implications for knowledge work

The Complex Needs work with its experience of providing Goldilocks Medicine for patients living with complex needs has helped me develop my own understanding of the 4Es elements of the knowledge work of generalist practice. But it has also provided valuable learning opportunities to share with colleagues developing their own skills.

Both the patients and clinicians involved in this work valued the Goldilocks approach. Patients appreciated the opportunity for a 'thorough', person-centred assessment and understanding of their needs. Clinicians engaged in the work found it rewarding and motivating to re-engage with their professional understanding of person-centred, advanced generalist care. Not all the clinicians who tried this work found it professionally rewarding. Some preferred to focus instead on other roles in the GP professional portfolio. Running the Complex Needs project reminded me that not all GPs are the same

The Complex Needs project continued for 12 months. In that time, the work enabled a de-escalation of inappropriate medicalisation, patient confidence in self-management based on shared understanding and explanation, and reported improvement in health for daily living. Perhaps most of all, this work highlighted that advanced generalist practice is not defined, or indeed adequately supported, by some of the traditional aspects of general practice. Generalist care needs more than 10-minute consultations backed up by the safety net of a continuing relationship with the GP. Instead, we need to recognise, respect and value the complexity of the work involved.

3.3 HEATH'S GENERALIST GATEKEEPER OR GURU

There is a common theme in the two examples I have described so far. Etz's concept of prioritisation is perhaps the most useful way to describe this work – the work of 'generalist triage'. The GP, with access to both specialist and advanced generalist skills, in 'sorting, ranking and negotiating' is looking to identify when the problem being presented needs more than a 'simple' biomedical understanding, but something more complex. In her Harveian lecture, in 2011, Iona Heath described this as the Gatekeeper role of the medical generalist (Heath 2011). But her account of what is involved is very different to traditional understanding of the GP gatekeeping role.

Within UK healthcare, patients can generally only access specialist healthcare through two routes: accident and emergency or by referral from general practice. The GP referral process has long acted to both 'filter' who accesses secondary healthcare, as well as guiding where people are seen. Under this traditional view of gatekeeping, the GP 'filters' out clear cases of disease which can easily be managed in primary care. People referred to secondary care are those who need advanced specialist care, or where the diagnosis is unclear and it is felt specialist assessment to rule in or out diagnosis could be helpful. In modern UK settings, the decision making in these referral processes are increasingly guided by (deductive reasoning based) care pathways which create criteria for 'access' to care.

Sripa et al. (2019) have reviewed the benefits to the healthcare system of this view of the GP 'gatekeeper to specialist care' role. In their Cochrane systematic review, which included 25 studies from around the world, they found that gatekeeping to specialist care was associated with reduced use of secondary care, but increased primary care visits. Quality of care (reported in terms of disease care outcomes) was generally higher where gatekeeping was present (with a possible exception related to cancer referrals); but patient satisfaction was lower. Like all reviews, this work was a critical analysis of existing published research, and therefore is a distillation of what has happened, and been researched, in the past. Healthcare systems in the UK and elsewhere are changing rapidly, including in the way that traditional 'gatekeeping' happens. We have seen new pathways for referral with changing use of screening tools, artificial intelligence and multiple health professionals involved in deciding which patients should gain access to specialist care. Therefore, we should not assume that Sripa's review findings can be applied with confidence to the new models of care now in place (and indeed Sripa called for new research). But evidence to date suggests that gatekeeping benefits secondary care services.

In her Harveian lecture, Heath described a different understanding of the Gatekeeper role – a Generalist Gatekeeper. A traditional understanding of gatekeeping recognises it is deciding whether an individual

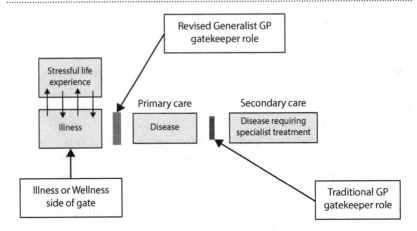

Figure 3.2   Heath's revised model of the Generalist Gatekeeper role. (Adapted from Heath 2011.)

can be managed in primary care or needs referral to advanced specialist (hospital-based) care (see Figure 3.2). Heath's new offering was to recognise the Generalist Gatekeeper role in assessing whether an individual may benefit from medicalisation of their illness experience.

Heath recognised that at any point in time, there will be a pool of people in a given community experiencing a disruption in their daily living that they perceive to be health, or illness, related. Many of these people will manage this illness themselves. I have already discussed the creative capacity and wider determinants that may shape their capacity to cope. Some people will bring their illness problem to the primary care practitioner: perhaps because they perceive they have a disease needing medical treatment, or because they are unsure about, or overwhelmed, by the illness and need advice or support to explore and explain what is happening. The Gatekeeper role of the Generalist, as described by Heath, is to recognise who has an illness that would benefit (in terms of optimising health for daily living) from medicalisation and intervention. But also to recognise the individuals for whom medicalisation of their illness experience may offer more harm than benefit. These people are best supported to deal with their illness experience in a non-medical approach. This is a very different understanding of the Gatekeeper role to that traditionally talked about in terms of referral to hospital care.

The Generalist Gatekeeper role involves the clinician in the tailored care and knowledge work I have been describing so far. The clinical question changes from a deductive approach, asking can I medicalise this illness problem (does the individual meet the criteria for a diagnosis), or an inductive one, asking should I medicalise this illness.

Once again, a case study will help to describe this. Let me introduce you to Hilda – another of my fictional patients based on real people I have worked with in practice over many years. Hilda has had three 'beyond target' blood pressure readings and so was flagged to see her GP to discuss risk management and medication. In this scenario, Hilda has been identified as 'sick' and in need of medical intervention – in Heath's model (Figure 3.2), she has passed from the 'illness' box to the 'disease' box. We know that management of blood pressure can reduce Hilda's risk of developing cardiovascular disease in the future. From a single disease perspective, 'medicalising' Hilda's illness into a 'disease' was the right decision for Hilda and the health service.

Each time Hilda is seen in practice, someone checks her blood pressure. Each time, it is 'off target'. So, following guideline care, the clinical team add in more medicines to better control Hilda's blood pressure. By the time I see her, she is on four tablets. Hilda has recently missed a number of routine check-up appointments at the practice. This was flagged to me as part of our Complex Needs work, and I go to see her at home to see how she's doing and undertake a whole person, generalist assessment of her health and healthcare needs.

The bottom line is that Hilda hasn't been taking any of the tablets she was given. She told me she didn't want to be labelled as 'ill'. She would far rather manage her health in other ways (Hilda describes that she eats well and goes out for a walk every day). 'I'll take my chances,' she says. But Hilda didn't know how to say that to the clinical team at the practice. She found it easier to collect the tablets (so we thought she was 'complying') but not take them. I removed several carrier bags of medicines from her house after our visit.

Hilda had rejected the transition from the 'illness/wellness' box to the 'disease' box. It wasn't incorrect to offer her the choice of 'moving over'. But in medicalising her risk (creating a new 'disease') we hadn't adequately explored Hilda's own understanding and perception of her health needs, her priorities for care and her thoughts on the impact of healthcare on her work for daily living. For Hilda, and from the perspective of maintaining her health for daily living, she preferred to stay on the non-medical side of the disease gate. She didn't think we as her healthcare team would understand that, so she opted out of seeing us at all.

Following a generalist discussion with Hilda, exploring her health needs in the context of her daily living, we agreed to review and revise the 'problem list' on her medical record – and so remove the 'diagnosis' of hypertension. Hilda had plans for reviewing her diet and lifestyle that would likely benefit her cardiovascular risk. By working with Hilda to explore and explain her health needs in this way, we reduced the burden of healthcare work for Hilda as she no longer had to pick up and pretend to take medication, and dread being called for a blood pressure review. This allowed her to focus instead on the work of daily living. The benefits to the practice were in avoiding wasteful prescribing (Ridge 2021) and time spent 'chasing' Hilda.

Heath's contribution was a radical re-assertion of the GP role. By clearly describing the generalist GP role to shift the question from *can* I diagnose this individual, to *should* I diagnose this individual, she gives permission for the generalist (beyond guideline) clinical approach. Her account recognised best practice as defined not by the ability to 'correctly' diagnose a patient, but to explore and explain whether it is in their best interests to do so.

This is a far more nuanced and complex understanding of the generalist clinician role than the 'jack of all trades' account – doing the simple bits and passing on the more complex elements to others. Gatekeeper is perhaps the wrong term for the work too – suggesting it is a simple yes or no, in or out approach to assessing and managing need. The 'gatekeeper' label for professional practice has long been challenged for its association with 'policing' something. Perhaps we should draw instead on Etz's description of a Prioritisation role – an action that is more about guidance than gatekeeping?

Patients have a growing access to information that enables them to understand for themselves if they meet the criteria for a disease condition. But understanding whether that diagnosis will help with the disruption to daily living they are experiencing is more nuanced. Take, for example, menopause. There has been a big public campaign in the UK to raise awareness and understanding of menopause and treatment options. I am seeing a growing number of patients wanting to explore HRT as an option for management of their health-related disruption to daily living. But for the majority of these people, there are many other factors involved, meaning that HRT alone is unlikely to provide the 'solution' they seek. That is not to suggest we shouldn't try, but we also need to work with individuals to help them understand and explain the full range of their illness experience; including what we will do if HRT alone doesn't work. The risk otherwise is that we cycle round using ever-higher doses of medication, and changing brands of medication, without ever meeting the healthcare needs of the individual. By asking the wrong question at the assessment process (not, *can* I diagnose this woman as menopausal, but *should* I diagnose this woman), we create additional burden both for our patients and the healthcare system.

There are a number of factors which now contribute to effectively 'bypass' the Generalist Gatekeeper function that Heath described. I have already mentioned some – including the widespread access to online diagnostic assessment tools, and the implementation of healthcare 'guidelines'. The introduction of digital triage tools may further exacerbate the problem. As I described, Gatekeeper might not be the right term for this role – perhaps we should rename the role as a Generalist Guru. But we urgently need to restore the function it served if we are to tackle the problems being created by transactional based healthcare systems that seek to improve diagnostic 'accuracy' but without sufficient attention to effectiveness in optimising health for daily living.

3.4 SUMMARY

In this chapter, I have described and discussed the knowledge work done by health professionals to enable tailored, whole person, generalist healthcare. I have highlighted that it is grounded in scientific practice – the systematic generation of knowledge (or trusted belief) which goes beyond the biomedical account of evidence-based medicine to support the flexibility needed for tailored whole person healthcare narratives. I have explored some of the tools that we can use to help generate tailored explanations, including the Flipped Consultation and using travelling consultations, to support the generation of tailored explanations. I have recognised that this approach can help address the daily challenges faced by patients in dealing with the burden of illness and healthcare, by clinicians overwhelmed by the burden of need and by health systems burdened by both demand and iatrogenic harm.

Yet in these accounts, I have repeatedly recognised the importance of context in shaping, supporting and undermining the knowledge work of daily practice. This is the theme I will explore in the next chapter.

REFERENCES

Barnett K et al. (2012). Epidemiology of multimorbidity and implications for health, research and medical education: A cross sectional study. Lancet, 380, pp. 37–43.

Engel G. (1977). The need for a new medical model: A challenge for biomedical science. Science, 196, pp. 126–129.

Etz R, Miller W, Stange K. (2021). Simple rules that guide generalist and specialist care. Family Medicine, 53(8), pp. 697–99.

Gut E. (1989). Productive and Unproductive Depression. London: Routledge.

Heath I. (2011). Divided we fail. Clinical Medicine Journal, 11(6), pp. 576–586.

Hughes L, McMurdo MET, Guthrie B. (2013). Guidelines for people not diseases: The challenges of applying UK clinical guidelines to people with multimorbidity. Age Aging, 42, pp. 62–69.

Lucassen P et al. (2018). Feeling blue, sad or depressed: how to manage these patients. BJGP, 68, p. 331.

Neighbour R. (2005). The Inner Consultation: How to Develop an Effective and Intuitive Consulting Style. London: Radcliffe Publishing.

Oakley A. (1989). Smoking in pregnancy: Smokescreen or risk factor? Sociology of Health and Illness, 11, pp. 311–334.

Reeve J. (2019). Unlocking the creative capacity of the self. In Dowrick C (Ed), Person-Centred Primary Care. Searching for the Self. Oxon: Routledge.

Ridge K. (2021). National overprescribing review report. Department of Health and Social Care, UK Government.

Rosendal M et al. (2017). "Medically unexplained" symptoms and symptoms disorders in primary care: Prognosis-based recognition and classification. BMC Family Practice, 18, p. 18.

Sripa P et al. (2019). Impact of GP gatekeeping on quality of care and health outcomes, use and expenditure: A systematic review. British Journal of General Practice, 69, pp. e294–303.

Swinglehurst D. (2019). Challenges to the 'self' in IT-mediated health care. In Dowrick C. (Ed), Person-Centred Primary Care. Searching for the Self. Oxon: Routledge.

CHAPTER 4

Wise places: Practices supporting expert generalist knowledge work

....

In this chapter, I turn to the consideration of Wise Places – the organisation of practice and how it enables or undermines the delivery of generalist, whole person healthcare.

4.1 ENABLING THE KNOWLEDGE WORK OF ADVANCED GENERALIST PRACTICE: REDESIGNING THE GENERALIST PRACTICE

Chapter 3 focused on the work of advanced generalist practice in the context of a consultation with an individual patient. That work happens in a wider context – the setting of a general practice. There are many other settings in which generalist care happens – including the broader wider primary care context and in secondary care. But I start with the GP surgery as the place in which I will develop our understanding of the knowledge work for generalist care. For readers working in other places, I look forward to hearing your thoughts on how these observations fit with, challenge, or indeed overlook key elements of the issues and challenges in your own workplaces.

Once again, I will use three case studies to illuminate the issues around place and generalist practice. For each case study, I will start with a brief description of what we did. I then turn to the specific knowledge work lessons arising from each case – with a particular focus on the implications for designing spaces – places for advanced generalist practice. At the end of the chapter, I conclude with a consideration of the common

DOI: 10.1201/9781003297222-4

threads arising from these examples and so the implications for primary care redesign.

4.2 BOUNCEBACK: ENABLING KNOWLEDGE WORK IN CONTEXT

In Chapter 3, I described our work to create a new generalist consultation approach for managing mild-moderate distress presenting in primary care. The Flipped Consultation model helps practitioners and patients to explore and potentially explain common mental health problems presenting in practice on the 'illness' (or non-biomedical) side of the medicalisation 'Gate' described by Iona Heath. Initial support focuses on an individual's social and psychological needs, with medicalisation considered only if problems persist.

There is experiential and research evidence to support the use of an alternative Flipped Consultation approach. Public, professional and policy voices have all expressed concern about the overmedicalisation of some mental health issues, leading – for example – to potentially suboptimal use of antidepressant medication. But there are some very real practical issues involved in trying to change the way that health services work. If we want to change clinical practice, we also need to look at – and potentially change – the context in which that work happens. This was the focus of the wider BOUNCEBACK project.

BOUNCEBACK grew from a conversation more than 10 years ago between a mental health charity (AiW Health), local GPs and university partners. All recognised that much of the mental health issues they were seeing on a daily basis had links and origins in concerns that were far wider than those addressed by pharmaceutical or even psychological (cognitive behavioural therapy) interventions. These discussions were happening before the formal introduction of social prescribing in the UK NHS, but can perhaps be understood as a precursor to that approach. Local practices were keen to understand how they could access that support for their patients.

AiW Health had many years of experience of using a Flipped Consultation approach to supporting the needs of local people experiencing distress. Their work had demonstrated the value and importance of first tackling the contextual (social and psychological) factors contributing to people's experiences. Only if distress persisted after this were people encouraged to contact their GP (consider a biomedical assessment).

And so we identified a question – would it be possible to embed AiW Health with their socio-psycho-bio approach to addressing distress into general practices? Our intention was that patients would have direct access to the socio-psycho support they most often needed, with biomedical backup from GPs available. We hoped to enable both demedicalisation of mild-moderate distress, whilst optimising the creative capacity of individuals; and enhancing the experience and outcomes for patients and clinicians alike. Our suggestion was that this change in approach to managing distress in the primary care setting could potentially contribute to improved mental health and health for daily living. This, in turn, could lead to reduced repeat health service use, altered prescribing, enhanced quality of life and strengthened personal and social capital.

Changing the whole model of, and approach to, primary mental healthcare was clearly an ambitious plan. Our first step therefore was to ask simply was small change possible? We set out to understand if and how we could embed new ways of working, and new teams into the general practice setting. This was to be the BOUNCEBACK project. BOUNCEBACK was designed as a feasibility study – to critically examine if we could introduce change. It wasn't designed to give us detailed information about the impact of the new service – for example on consultation rates, re-attendance and prescribing. But we did collect case study data that helped us understand what was happening, why, and if and how it could be improved (see Box 4.1).

Here, I want to focus on what we learnt from doing the feasibility study. Designing, running and learning from BOUNCEBACK is an example of professional knowledge work in practice. It involved us in using the 4Es to generate, use and learn from knowledge work on the ground, but this time with a focus on changing practice, not just the clinical management of an individual patient. Through this work, we were able to identify three themes relevant to understanding how we can deliver change on the ground in general practice: the need for new Teams, new Triage and new Learning. I'll discuss each of these in turn. But first let's take a look at the knowledge work process itself.

Introducing normalisation process theory

I briefly mentioned Normalisation Process Theory (NPT) in Chapter 2 when I discussed barriers to generalist practice. NPT was developed by a team led by Professor Carl May based on extensive study of introducing and embedding change into practice settings. It is now widely used in healthcare research to help introduce change. All of which is why

BOX 4.1 SUMMARY OF EVALUATION FINDINGS FROM THE BOUNCEBACK PROJECT

The evaluation used a case study approach to address three questions:

Who did we deliver care to?

- The service was embedded into seven practices in NW England, of varying size.
- 247 patients were referred (by self or others) into the service and 69% attended their first appointment.
- 40% of the service users were men.

What service was delivered?

- We described a model of care based on the Flipped Consultation approach and a practice manual for delivery (see Reeve 2016).
- Average number of consultations per patient was 2.6.
- Evaluation revealed that the BOUNCEBACK approach was used, at least in part, in most of these consultations.

What outcomes were observed?

- To quote one service user: 'The service achieved its aim for me of offering an alternative and practical solution to medication'.
- People developed new understanding of their problems and health issues.
- The data collection processes for measuring quantitative outcomes (mental wellbeing and assessment of activity participation) unfortunately failed.

Full details are available in Reeve (2016).

we decided to use it to support our practice-based knowledge work for the BOUNCEBACK project.

Essentially, NPT tells us that if we want to embed a new way of working into everyday practice, we need to pay attention to four key elements. The full theory is more complex and nuanced than the summary I use in this chapter. If you're thinking about using NPT, I'd recommend that you explore the NPT website and read about it in more detail (May et al. n.d.). For BOUNCEBACK, we focused on a less detailed version that still recognises the core components of NPT. This recognised that if we wanted to embed the BOUNCEBACK approach into everyday practice, we would need to pay attention to four elements: Sense making, Engagement, Action and Monitoring. The new way of working must make sense to the people using and doing the work – so they understand what is trying to do, why and how it can benefit them. People need to be able to engage with the work – start doing it and continue the work. Not everyone comes onboard at the same time (or indeed at all). People must have the skills and resources to be able to do (Action) the work. They must also receive feedback that enables and supports them to continue the work – to observe and monitor the effect of their actions. It is probably already apparent that these four elements overlap, and indeed May acknowledges this within his discussions of NPT. For example, it is only possible for workers to engage with a new work of working if they understand what it is and why it matters. Nonetheless the four areas provide a useful framework for planning, and monitoring change. We used this framework to help us design how we were going to implement BOUNCEBACK, and also to help us monitor and learn from the work on the ground.

Setting up BOUNCEBACK

Our goal was to introduce and use the Flipped Consultation approach for dealing with distress presenting to general practice where no red flags (risks) were identified. Our plan was to introduce AiW-trained BOUNCEBACK case workers into seven local GP practices to deliver care. Patients registered at the GP practices would be able to book directly with the BOUNCEBACK case workers. Reception staff signposted patients to the new service. Patients who presented to GPs or practice nurses with problems that included distress could also be internally referred.

Case workers used a socio-psycho-bio approach to explore, understand and so manage patient needs. AiW case workers were able to access resources and supports outside of the NHS where appropriate to help with non-biomedical issues (e.g., help with finance, benefits, housing, skills, work, social contacts). The case workers arranged repeat follow-up with the patients for as long as was necessary. Any concerns that couldn't be addressed by the BOUNCEBACK worker were referred back to the GP.

Embedded within the BOUNCEBACK project was an evaluation team overseeing the design, delivery and learning from the set-up of the service. We planned to use a Trial and Learn approach not just in our clinical consultations with patients, but also in our whole team approach to implement a new way of working.

The team used NPT to design a traffic light system to monitor the actions, and impact, of work in each of the four areas of work that NPT predicted would be needed for this project to work. Members of the core BOUNCEBACK team (including AiW, practice teams and researchers) met on a monthly basis to review process and progress against each of the four elements of Sense Making, Engagement, Action and Monitoring. This allowed us to explore what was working well, what barriers we were experiencing, and what we needed to do to overcome them. As we set up BOUNCEBACK and started running the service, we hit many snags – both expected and unexpected. For example, we anticipated that local communities would be slow to take up and trust a new service and we certainly saw this. However, we also soon discovered we had underestimated the work we would need to do with practice teams as well. Most of the challenges we hit in setting up the new service were related to knowledge work issues and these are the ones I will focus on here.

Essentially, our key learning points were that we needed to rethink our understanding of *Access*; recognise and engage an Extended *Team*; and alter the goal of practice to a focus on *Learning*.

Generalist care: Reconsidering access

We designed two access points into the BOUNCEBACK service: patients could book directly with a case worker, or be referred by their GP or other member of the clinical team. As we had anticipated, patients used (engaged with) both approaches. However, what we had underestimated was how the choice of access route would impact the process of Exploration of a patient's problem and so the Explanation generated through consultation. This, in turn, impacted how patients were able to engage with the BOUNCEBACK approach and so the outcomes of care. Let me describe what we observed.

Patients who came into BOUNCEBACK from their GP had often already had a biopsychosocial consultation with a clinician to explore their problem. In these cases, people arrived with an already formed biomedical explanation of their illness experience (e.g. as a neurotransmitter imbalance in their brain requiring medication). These patients told us that they were either unsure why they had been referred to BOUNCEBACK, or expecting that they were there to 'receive a service' (for example, specific help with their finances). In these circumstances, the case workers reported finding it more difficult to use a Flipped Consultation approach and engage those patients in discussions of alternative approaches to understanding and addressing their distress. It became clear that we needed to think more broadly about the question of how people 'access' a service – including the impact of that process on their understanding and expectations of the healthcare service.

In the NHS, we commonly conflate the issues of 'access' and 'availability'. We monitor the quality of healthcare using 'access' measures such as waiting times. We defend criticism of general practice access by describing the number of appointments per month that are available and used by patients (currently 33 million per month in England). Both waiting times, and number of appointments are measures of availability of a service, but not necessarily of *access* – at least if we recognise access as a broader concept of 'helping people to command healthcare resources in order to preserve or improve their health' (Gulliford et al. 2002).

Our experiences in the BOUNCEBACK project showed us that it wasn't enough to just make the service available to people by putting case workers into the practice setting – we also had to make it accessible. Kovandžić et al. (2011) offer a useful framework to think about how we do that. Based on an analysis of data from multiple research studies examining issues of access, Kovandžić proposed that to help people 'command healthcare resources', we need to pay attention to three elements: candidacy, concordance and recursivity.

Candidacy is a concept first developed by Dixon-Woods et al. (2006). Essentially, for someone to approach and seek help from healthcare, they need to recognise themselves as a suitable 'candidate' for care. Candidacy therefore refers to the processes by which people understand whether they are eligible to use a service. Concordance relates to the factors which shape the capacity for shared working between patient and clinician. This is the development of shared understanding of the explanation of the problem and resources available to manage it. Recursivity describes how contact with healthcare services shapes an individual's future healthcare-seeking behaviour – have we left this individual better able to deal with a similar problem in the future?

Advanced generalist approaches, including the Flipped Consultation, can potentially help with both concordance and recursivity. BOUNCEBACK experiences led us to recognise we also needed to focus more on the element of 'candidacy'. We needed to re-consider the pathways by which people came to the service, including how these experiences shaped their ideas about what care they needed. Because we were using NPT to monitor the implementation of this new service in real time, we were able to introduce changes to how we worked with the whole practice team to tackle this issue. I'll talk more about that shortly.

Some patients rejected the BOUNCEBACK approach. We saw several stories like that of Tom, a young man who described that he was finding it difficult to cope with lots of things going on. He didn't have a job and was struggling with his benefits and finances. The Jobcentre staff were 'pushing' him to apply for jobs but he felt he was not well enough to be applying for jobs. He felt anxious and overwhelmed a lot of the time. He admitted he was drinking quite a bit to cope, often on his own as he was socially isolated. He had fallen out with his family. Tom felt he needed antidepressants to help with his mood and to be signed off as not fit for work. When we tried using a Flipped Consultation approach with Tom, he became angry and stormed out of the consulting room – angry with our exploration approach and certainly nowhere near a shared 'explanation' to support a concordant working partnership. Many clinicians will have met a 'Tom'. In the context of the BOUNCEBACK project, we were left reflecting on the potential need to rethink our 'front door' to general practice – how we engage with communities, public sector partners and more – to develop a better shared understanding of what general practice can, and can't, offer. I'll return to this point in Chapter 6.

Generalist care: A whole team approach

As I have highlighted, access issues also prompted us to reflect on the need to recognise a whole team approach to delivery of whole person care.

I mentioned that AiW case workers often struggled to engage patients with the BOUNCEBACK approach if they had already been given a biomedical explanation for their distress by their GP. We therefore decided we needed to work with those GPs to help them understand the Flipped Consultation method too. GPs obviously remained free to use whatever clinical approach they thought was appropriate in their consultations. Our intention was simply to offer them greater understanding of the BOUNCEBACK work to support access issues related to both candidacy and concordance. So we invited clinicians at BOUNCEBACK practices to understand the flipped approach to help them both recognise patients who may benefit from referral to a BOUNCEBACK worker, and to help them start patients to explore their understanding of their distress.

A case may help me describe this better. Let us imagine that Helen comes in to see her GP, Dr Smith, in a BOUNCEBACK practice. Dr Smith has been on the Flipped Consultation course and so feels able to use these approaches to start a conversation with Helen. It quickly becomes clear that Helen is currently navigating very choppy waters, with very limited ballast and support (see Chapter 1). Dr Smith reflects back to Helen that she sounds exhausted. Helen immediately bursts into tears and agrees. At this point, Dr Smith suggests that dealing with this exhaustion might be an important starting point for helping Helen, and introduces her to the BOUNCEBACK worker in her practice. Helen agrees to try working with them.

By having shared understanding of the purpose and value of a BOUNCEBACK approach within the primary care team, Dr Smith is able to help Helen explore and engage with the approach. Helen recognises herself a 'candidate' for this service and is able to book time to spend with a case worker to explore the possibilities to work together on the problem. Helen goes to see the case worker a number of times to have the space to explore, develop explanations and ways forward and to follow up and evaluate the effect of these approaches. Dr Smith is able to deal with a range of other patient needs. We have potentially improved Helen's access to effective care as well as Dr Smith's availability to deliver accessible care to others. Achieving this meant integrating the BOUNCEBACK (generalist) approach into the wider primary care team.

Generalist care: Changing the goal

BOUNCEBACK sought to deliver a different model of healthcare. We weren't just bringing case workers into practice to provide more capacity to do the same thing. We wanted to change the model of practice: to engage patients and clinicians in a different understanding of their distress, and therefore a different approach to managing it. We aimed to work with individuals to co-create a new understanding of their illness experience and so of how they might, with support, deal with it. We aimed to change three elements of the way people access healthcare – candidacy, concordance and recursivity – through enhancing the creative capacity of an individual using the Flipped Consultation approach to help create new understanding and action. The model sought to enhance the capacity of individuals and communities to be part of improving their health. Exploration, making sense and creating understanding was foregrounded as an integral part of care. This work was therefore something to be prioritised and resourced within the healthcare setting (e.g., in the design of consultation spaces and lengths).

Evaluating and demonstrating the impact of those changes on broader healthcare outcomes was an aspect of learning that we struggled to introduce into our service redesign. Routine data collection was insufficient to capture the processes and outcomes of the new model of care. We had external researchers supporting the implementation and evaluation of the new service, but TO COLLECT the day-to-day data NEEDED to demonstrate the impact of the service WE needed – the involvement of staff on the ground. This sort of activity is not built into their routine everyday work and so, not surprisingly, we failed to capture that data.

Theory, and some initial data, supports an understanding that the Flipped Consultation approach in the BOUNCEBACK model can be implemented in practice, and may support positive changes for patients and practitioners alike (including deprescribing, and enhanced capacity for self-management). However, it also showed us that if we want to make practice-level changes, we needed to build practice-level monitoring and learning approaches into the new models of care. We needed to prioritise the new data and analysis processes involved to support the generation of (practice-level) knowledge-in-context. We needed to move towards a learning organisation model of care.

Generalist care: Towards a learning organisation

UK general practice prides itself on delivering care the communities it serves. The work that they do is heavily dictated by external sources. Contractual mechanisms describe the units of care they are expected to provide, dictated largely by externally described guidelines for best practice. But UK general practice is also recognised for its ability to respond quickly and innovatively to change. In recent years, it has been able to respond rapidly to a host of changes: workforce challenges, leading to the introduction of new members of practice teams; service delivery requirements, with the greater use of digital technology; and changing service models (e.g., the introduction of new providers including social prescribing). The recent Fuller (2022) report discussing Next Steps for General Practice describes many examples of practices delivering innovation in service delivery.

But the BOUNCEBACK project duplication highlighted that change, certainly sustained change, needs more than just a good idea. BOUNCEBACK was an example of primary care teams delivering clinical innovation. But innovation is not just about adding something – bolting on a new way of working into an existing setting – it also involves the introduction of new skills and approaches across a whole community of practice. Whole teams need access to resources that enable them to explore, explain and evaluate (review and revise) new ways of working on the ground.

The 'trial and learn' approach described in the knowledge work of patient care also applies to the practice-level knowledge work needed to successfully introduce and embed change and new ways of working. BOUNCEBACK highlighted that we needed to recognise general practice not just as a setting in which practice is delivered (rules are followed), but a critical, creative space in which knowledge and information is created, used and adapted in context to generate new learning for context (see also Chapter 2). Achieving change to deliver advanced generalist models of care needs the support of practices designed as learning organisations. I will return to this theme in Chapter 6.

Generalist care: In summary

BOUNCEBACK was a whole-practice example of the implementation and use of knowledge work on the ground. It highlighted the use of the 4Es to drive change enabling whole person, generalist care for patients and communities. It demonstrated that knowledge work needs a clear FRAMEWORK to provide SAFE BOUNDARIES that support the critical, creative knowledge work of practice (in this case the principles of the Flipped Consultation and the Exhaustion Cycle). It requires us to create a clear and supported SPACE for the knowledge work needed, including the critical reflection and learning that enables individuals and teams to undertake this knowledge work. It needs a TEAM approach with changes in the way we design practices to provide the necessary time, resources, permission and prioritisation within the 'day job'. I will return to these at end of this chapter.

4.3   COMPLEX NEEDS: ENABLING KNOWLEDGE WORK IN CONTEXT FOR MULTIMORBIDITY

In Chapter 3, I described the Goldilocks Medicine consultation – the clinical work needed to optimise whole person care. I recognised that this model of care is complex and potentially resource intensive. I suggested that the approach may be particularly useful for those at greatest risk of harm from overmedicalisation – for example those living with complex multimorbidity. That consultation approach grew out of a broader Quality Improvement project that I led a few years ago. The Complex Needs project ran as an 18-month Quality Improvement project aiming to provide Goldilocks care to around 100 patients based at a single practice in Northwest England. That project allowed us to look critically at the practicality of delivering Goldilocks medicine in everyday care, and so consider what, if anything, needed to change in the way we design and run practices to enable this work. From the Complex Needs project, I identified some key elements that we need to take forward to our consideration of how to redesign primary care practice

Introducing the Complex Needs project

A few years ago, I was working in an inner-city practice in a deprived area. Like many practices, we had a group of patients on our practice list who were housebound and also living with multiple long-term conditions. These people included some of the most clinically vulnerable patients registered with us. We had good systems in place to visit these patients for an annual health check – a routine check or monitoring of things like their blood pressure, blood tests and medication. But for many of these people, the only GP visits they had were for urgent visits when they were acutely unwell. These acute, on the day, visits weren't usually geared towards a whole person, expert generalist review of health for daily living. There was no time for a proactive, whole person review of healthcare needs, priorities and planning. The practice team were concerned about unmet healthcare needs within this group of housebound patients.

So we decided to do something about it. There were local initiatives at the time to free up funding for innovative projects. We decided to use our funding to create some dedicated GP time to proactively visit, assess and address the whole person needs of this group of patients. The project was set up as a Quality Improvement project, asking: What is the impact of creating dedicated time for whole person assessment and management of healthcare needs for people who are housebound and living with multiple long-term conditions? The Complex Needs project (Box 4.2) allowed us to put Goldilocks Medicine into practice and learn from the effect. I have already discussed the clinical, patient-level knowledge work for this in Chapter 3. Here, I want to look at the practice-level changes and what we learned from them.

Developing the complex needs project

We knew we wanted to introduce a whole person assessment of illness for our vulnerable housebound population; producing tailored care plans that aimed to enhance, certainly not underline, health for daily living. But where and how should we start?

BOX 4.2 DESCRIBING THE COMPLEX NEEDS PROJECT

This 18-month Quality Improvement project was funded by Neighbourhood Efficiency Savings to deliver 1.5 days/week of GP time for this work.

WHO: People registered with the practice coded as homeless with 3+ long-term conditions on their problem list, 5+ medicines a day and record of unplanned medical admissions in the last year.

WHAT WE DID:

Clinical work: Clinical record review to identify current illness and treatment work/burden, contextual data were available. Dedicated home visit (45–60 min) for whole person review of goals, current care, opportunities for change and management plan. A management plan was added to patient record to support continuity of approach across a team. Follow-up was as determined by individual need.

Learning work: Using routine recorded data to describe what we did and the impact; discussed with the practice team to decide future work.

HOW WE DID IT:

Clinical work: Implementing Goldilocks Medicine through use of the advanced generalist skills from Chapter 2 to explore, explain and evaluate the impact of illness and change.

Learning work: Use of the same scholarship skills to collect and interpret data to explain the impact of the change and so describe the implications for ongoing delivery.

IMPACT:

Practice team recognition of the significance and value of expert generalist capacity for managing complex care; data provided some early signals suggesting improved outcomes for patients; demonstrating the need for further critical review and learning to guide future practice. The TAILOR project (see Chapter 5) was one piece of work to come out of this project.

There were no reported safety incidents or adverse events during the 9 months of the project.

For further details, see Reeve and Bancroft (2014).

Initially, the team recognised a few basic questions: who were we going to see, who was going to see them, what were they going to do, how they would record and share that with the team, and how we would evaluate what we'd done? These gave us a starting point. Essentially, we created a register of patients we thought were most at risk of needing a different approach: people who were housebound, living with three or more long-term conditions and five or more medicines. This work took place before practices routinely held coded frailty scores for our older patients, so used the best information we had at the time. We didn't set age limits for our new service. At the time, the practice had around 7,000 registered patients. Of these, around 100 patients met our criteria for the Complex Needs work. All members of the GP team could also refer new patients to the team if they were concerned, and the patient met our eligibility criteria.

We had funding for about 1.5 days GP time per week for about 9 months. We invited all interested GPs in the practice to be part of the work. After trying things out, there were two of us who were regularly doing this work. On average, the two GPs would see around eight patients a day. A first assessment took around 90 minutes in total including notes review, travel time and visits to explore and start to create a tailored explanation of healthcare needs. This time included the work to record and action management plans. Follow-up visits were at the discretion of the Complex Needs GPs – determined by the needs for further face to face evaluation of tailored care plans. Some people on the Complex Needs list needed just one visit to re-focus existing care plans. Follow-up was then provided through the routine reviews already offered in the practice. Other patients needed an ongoing tailored approach.

We reorganised the working week of clinicians in the practice to enable the knowledge work of tailored healthcare – the processes of exploration, explanation and evaluation. This required a reprioritisation of work for those clinicians, stepping away from 'standard' practice to offer a tailored service to a prioritised group.

Evaluation of the Complex Needs approach was built into the new model of working from the outset. The two GPs involved met to discuss cases and offer cross support. We also met with community matrons, and worked with the local consultant in community geriatrician and her team to discuss both individual patient needs, and the running of the project. As the project was funded by local practice efficiency savings, we also had to provide feedback to the funders on the impact and learning from the project.

Our initial project question asked: What is the impact of creating dedicated time for whole person assessment and management of healthcare needs for people who are housebound and living with multiple long-term conditions? Based on our evaluation of the first stage of the Complex Needs project, we found that most patients and staff liked the new way of working; but not everyone 'benefited' from the alternative model of practice.

Almost all patients liked the new service – having a proactive visit from a GP, at a time when they were not necessarily feeling poorly, in order to discuss their on-going health and care needs. Some were initially suspicious about the motivation for the visit, but few refused care. Practice staff also appreciated the benefits of the project. The Complex Needs offer provided a safety net for clinicians expressed concerns about missing unmet needs for this complex group of patients. The practice team valued the support and back up offered to the whole team in providing additional resource for managing complex problems, and improving the clarity and sharing of management plans for this complex group. Patient satisfaction is widely recognised as a marker of healthcare quality, and patients verbally reported high levels of satisfaction with the care. Staff satisfaction is also crucial for workforce morale and motivation, and hence to healthcare quality. The positive impact of the project on staff morale was also important. But those funding this work wanted to know that the patients received more than just a 'nice visit' that they 'liked'. Indeed funders, and service delivery staff alike, needed to know whether the approach supported clinically significant and meaningful changes to care.

This was a Quality Improvement project, not a research project. We had limited resource to collect new data to evaluate, and learn from, the new care – beyond our observations with patients. We relied on an analysis of routine data to help us explore, and seek to explain, the changes we saw. We noted that many of the changes resulting from the re-exploration and explanation of healthcare needs in this patient group related to the use of long-term diagnoses and medication. I described Hilda's experience of care in Chapter 3. Through the use of the knowledge work skills of exploration and explanation, Hilda agreed with her GP that management of cardiovascular risk was not a priority and she chose to discontinue her hypertensive medicines, and remove a diagnostic code of 'Essential Hypertension'.

We used this observation to help us look deeper into the routine clinical data that we were collecting. The two clinicians involved in this work noted that whilst we were making clinically significant changes in care plans for some patients, for others these visits largely just supported some 'clinical housekeeping' – tidying up of clinical records and coding in patients who were stable and managing their daily lives well. We decided to explore this more and look to see if there were any differences that might explain why someone was in the 'stable' group or the 'change' group. We understood the 'stable' group to be those for whom routine chronic disease(specialist) management (largely protocol driven) was sufficient to support daily living. The 'change' group were those for whom routine specialist care was contributing to vulnerability and risk of disruption to daily living.

Of the 100 patients on our register, about two-thirds were in the 'change group'. Goldilocks Medicine had led to clinically significant changes to the explanation and management plans being used to support their healthcare. This was a small population size so the potential for statistical analysis was limited, but there did not appear to be any statistically significant difference in biomedical parameters between the two groups: for example, no differences in the average number of long-term conditions or number of medicines between the groups. However, we did see some differences – we noted that people in the 'change' group were more likely to be experiencing one or more of three things: changes in their life circumstances (for example, moving into supported accommodations), mental health issues (including both mood and cognitive issues) or lack of social support (for example, being socially isolated). Each of these elements potentially impacts the creative capacity of individuals outlined in Chapter 1, and so their capacity to manage the work of chronic illness. The Complex Needs project highlighted both that we needed to recognise variability in the capacity of people living with long-term complex illness to manage their health issues, and to look beyond biomedical parameters to identify those at risk.

Evaluating the knowledge work involved

So did introducing dedicated time for the knowledge work needed to provide advanced generalist care to people living with long-term conditions who were housebound make a difference? Our conclusion was that yes it did – for some patients, and especially those with non-biomedically defined vulnerabilities creating reduced capacity for managing daily living. We also noted that the work brought benefit for staff: providing valuable support (capacity and headspace) for the wider team, together with improved job satisfaction and motivation for those involved. But introducing this way of working required significant changes in the way we organised the 'place' of care – the practice.

The Complex Needs project created ringfenced resources for the knowledge work of tailored healthcare. This enabled the team to PRIORITISE a complex patient group, it gave PERMISSION for clinicians to see and assess patients using a whole person medicine approach focused on addressing health as a resource for daily living and it provided additional opportunity and resources for the PERFORMANCE MONITORING of the impact of care that enabled individual clinicians, the practice team and indeed the wider community to learn from this model of practice.

The Complex Needs work highlighted the need for new and additional resources to support this work. Clinicians needed different data sets, including those linked to understanding creative capacity and resources for daily living as well as assessing biomedical demands on daily living. This finding flagged the importance of capacity for face-to-face reviews of patients, and therefore in this case for home visits to support exploration and the creation of explanation in context.

Clinicians also needed new resources to support the creation, sharing and review of whole person tailored care plans. Tailored care often involved working beyond standard guideline for care. Other members of the wider clinical team needed to understand how and why these changes had been implemented so they felt safe supporting and continuing them. This was particularly an issue for decisions related to prescribing, and this observation prompted the development of the TAILOR project that I will discuss in Chapter 5. We recognised that the way we design practice records, including the digital resources we use, to store and share clinical records needs to change.

The Complex Needs work highlighted the need for practice-level changes to support advanced generalist care. These included the need for new approaches to Access and Prioritisation of care. We initially prioritised housebound patients living with biomedically defined vulnerability to disruption to daily living. The Complex Needs work itself revealed that we need to also factor in wider, non-biomedical elements that affect creative capacity.

We also once again recognised the importance of working with practice *teams*. I have already recognised the importance of shared care planning to support consistent delivery of care. Shared working also offered an important source of support and safety netting for clinicians involved in what is often viewed as 'higher risk', beyond protocol care. Prioritised time for knowledge work also allowed for clearly defined lines of responsibility and accountability in the complex decision making involved in care for this group. But team working, and team reflection, was also seen to prompt a sense of professional satisfaction and pride across the team.

The Complex Needs project demonstrated that we can change the design of everyday practice work, but also that changes are needed if we are to deliver whole person, tailored care. Some of those changes resonated with the BOUNCEBACK work (for example, the importance of supporting teams in learning organisations); whilst some new findings were noted (for example, issues about safe boundaries and potential new roles for digital technology). I now consider my third case study before looking at the overall conclusions from this chapter.

4.4   PACT: CREATING PLACES FOR TAILORED CARE KNOWLEDGE WORK

In Chapter 3, I discussed how we can help professionals to practice differently to deliver advanced generalist care. But my research, and indeed my own clinical experience, has repeatedly highlighted that the context in which we work is crucially important in determining whether patients receive advanced generalist care. There is no point in changing the skills and approaches of clinicians if we don't also change the context in which they are working. This was brought home to me in the third of my case studies – the PACT initiative.

Introducing PACT

PACT (Patient-Aligned Care Team) was a UK primary care innovation project intended to deliver a new model of primary care support to people living with frailty and multimorbidity. A regional primary healthcare management team (known at the time in the UK as a Clinical Commissioning Group [CCG]) had recognised that standard disease-focused care wasn't meeting the needs of this patient group within their local populations Studies were repeatedly highlighting that people living with frailty and multiple long-term conditions were struggling with the double whammy of both disease and treatment burden. Local primary care leaders wanted to change the way care was being delivered to this vulnerable group.

The CCG therefore developed PACT – an evidence-informed new model of care targeting this group of people. The PACT 'toolkit' consisted of guidance on both identifying at risk patients (establishing a register of patients in need) and the use of the Comprehensive Geriatric Assessment tool to develop and record a tailored management plan for each individual. PACT was developed and rolled out on an understanding that the new model of care would need: additional staff and associated funding, new guidance on how to deliver care (the PACT toolkit) and new incentive payments for meeting set targets. Staff funding included protected time for a GP lead, funding for new nursing staff to deliver the guideline focused care and funding to support the administrative processes needed to record the new assessments and measure outcomes.

Of the 33 practices in the region, 32 signed up to deliver the new PACT service. Each practice was supported to develop a frailty register. PACT-funded Advanced Nurse Practitioners (ANPs) were offered a resource pack including the Geriatric Comprehensive Assessment toolkit to support initial assessment of patients on that list. Follow-up care was at the discretion of the clinical team in individual practices.

Evaluating PACT

The CCG were keen not only to deliver PACT, but to observe and learn from its impact. They wanted to understand what impact, if any, this enhanced service was having on the health and wellbeing of their local community. This would guide their decisions about whether to continue to fund, and potentially extend and expand, the PACT service. They therefore approached my team, working in the local academic primary care group, to evaluate the new service (Bryce et al. 2018).

The evaluation sought to understand what was being delivered and to consider the merit and worth (Stufflebeam 1973) of the new service. We used the NPT informed approaches that I have described elsewhere. We collected data on PACT through a variety of approaches so we could understand how PACT was working. These included observations of the PACT teams in action, interviews with practice staff and observation and discussion with CCG stakeholders and commissioners. We also invited all staff across the CCG – both those involved in delivering PACT and those that weren't – to share their views and thoughts through completing an NPT survey tool (Finch 2018). The researchers involved were experienced primary care scientists, but not clinicians.

Witnessing the knowledge work of daily practice

What we saw was the knowledge work of generalist, whole person, tailored healthcare. By observing, talking with and surveying patients and professionals, we explored how they worked to make sense of illness, and so to deliver tailored healthcare.

The staff involved in delivering the care were predominantly ANPs. These are experienced primary care clinicians who had been working with people living with chronic illness for many years. They brought a wealth of professional experience and expertise to consultations with the patients with frailty who were on their support lists. Most of them hadn't been using the tools included in the PACT toolkit, especially the Comprehensive Geriatric Assessment (CGA) tool, prior to the introduction of PACT. We saw mixed views on whether the CGA helped with the knowledge work of tailored practice. Some staff found using the consultation model a useful way to open up wider conversations with their patients – enabling the EXPLORATION of tailored practice. But others told us the CGA got in the way of their established professional practice and disabled EXPLORATION. But crucially, most of the staff reported that the CGA limited their ability to move from EXPLORATION to EXPLANATION. The tool was unable to support them in integrating patient and chronic disease narratives to generate a tailored EXPLANATION of illness. The CGA tool, as it was presented in the PACT initiative, helped them collect information, but not use it in a useful/meaningful way to offer tailored explanations of problems and so deliver personalised, whole person care.

The effect we observed in watching PACT in action was of enhanced exploration of illness in the context of daily living but without adequate support for generating new explanations. This led to a 'Pandora's box' scenario. Clinical assessment generated an ever longer list of potential or new problems, but with insufficient support to prioritise, interpret or action those issues. We observed staff teams finding themselves working harder and longer to try and address growing lists of long-standing problems and gaps, all without sufficient resource. There was clear evidence of risk of burnout within some of the teams.

In other teams, we noted staff with the experience and expertise to manage this information (over)load created by the enhanced exploration of need, and use it to create new tailored management plans for patients. This then created new challenges when the identified needs didn't map to the resources available to deal with them. Staff described initially welcoming a move to a more holistic approach to understanding and managing complex patient needs, only to be left feeling frustrated and overwhelmed. The tools and resources they had been offered for PACT didn't adequately help them to deliver whole person care. Indeed, in some cases, PACT hindered whole person care by creating burnout and overload.

In Chapter 2, I recognised that the construction of knowledge-in-context needs a clear vision of the goal of care to provide a framework of support for the critical creative knowledge work that follows. Our evaluation of PACT highlighted that that practice teams shared a vision of the value of whole person care and that this was present before the introduction of PACT. We also observed that the tools introduced as part of PACT – the GCA along with additional staff – enabled the whole person exploration of needs and problems faced by individual patients. But what we noted was lacking was the resources needed to translate findings from exploration into effective tailored explanations and management plans for individuals. There was a lack of capacity for the structured evaluation (review and revision) that is an integral part of defining quality of care in inductive, interpretive generalist practice. PACT once again emphasised the issue raised by the Complex Needs project, that staff need clear frameworks and safe boundaries to support delivery of complex care. These were missing in PACT, leaving staff feeling overwhelmed and burdened by revealed patient need; with no capacity to either address that need, or set legitimate boundaries on what could and couldn't be done.

Implications for practice redesign for knowledge work

PACT taught us a number of lessons about improving generalist care in context. Firstly, more of the same won't do. PACT gave teams more (new) tools, and more staff. But these resources were essentially intended to support a greater volume of the same type of activity: assessment of illness status and implementation of management plans.

PACT staff reported lacking both skills in the interpretive knowledge work needed for advanced generalist practice. They lacked confidence in the professional skills needed to produce and use tailored explanations of illness management for individuals, including knowing when to stop or de-escalate medical care. But implementing the PACT initiative also raised daily questions for staff that extended beyond clinical issues. Every stage in the process generated questions for front-line clinicians about how to run the PACT service. Who was eligible for care, and who should be prioritised? What health and healthcare needs were 'relevant' for the PACT service and what shouldn't (or couldn't) be covered? How long should people be followed up for following initial assessment – bearing in mind that the more people they had under review, the fewer new assessments they could take on. Implementing PACT generated real challenges for practice teams related to service design and delivery (including setting goals and prioritising care). This generated a significant amount of work for PACT teams. Yet, none of this work was recognised by, or funded for, within the service contract for delivering PACT.

PACT was an example of a complex intervention. As I described in Chapter 1, this is a model of care with multiple interacting parts; where the process of, and outcomes from, delivery cannot be predicted using simple linear pathways and algorithms. Our evaluation of PACT resonates with other case studies discussed in this chapter, highlighting that successful implement of these approaches into primary care needs inbuilt capacity for flexibility and adaptability. Practice teams therefore need inbuilt resources for, or access to expertise in, the knowledge work of generating understanding in context. This practice-level work can be described in terms of the same 4Es approach I have described – the critical creative processes involved in applied Epistemological action, Exploration, Explanation and Evaluation. Advanced generalist practitioners will have experience and expertise in these skills; but still require resources (including space) to apply them. But these skills are not automatically taught to all healthcare professionals, so we can't assume that practice teams will be able to do this work. Indeed, our evaluation of PACT demonstrated that many aren't able – with detrimental effects on staff wellbeing as a result.

PACT was valued by patients and professionals, but the lack of clarity on its aims was identified as a barrier to implementation. Contracts developed with PACT practices focused on service *delivery* outcomes, but not on the service *development* needed to achieve the goals. Implementation of new models of care in practice needs to be evidence-informed – supporting the knowledge work of innovation and change – rather than evidence-dictated.

4.5 CONCLUSIONS: CREATING WISE PLACES

In this chapter, I have presented case studies describing practice-level implementation of advanced generalist care. There are many overlaps between the three. Together they support the case for a number of specific actions needed to deliver advanced generalist practices – the Wise Places that support advanced generalist care in action.

To create Wise Places, we need to rethink how we understand ACCESS to healthcare. This includes how both patients and healthcare understand and recognise candidacy – eligibility for healthcare use; along with prioritisation of care. In Chapter 7, Stefan Hjorleiffson will mention work in Norway to 'renegotiate' the general practice contract with their communities. In Chapter 6, I will consider the need for a new 'front door' for general practice.

Wise Places need clearly described TEAMS. Teams contain the diversity of skills and knowledge needed for critical creative knowledge work action, and potentially provide the capacity to confidently support this work. But within those teams, we need people with clearly defined roles and links, including defined responsibilities and boundaries.

Advanced generalist practice – whether at the level of individual patient care, or running a practice-level service – is inherently uncertain. Individuals and teams need clear frameworks providing safe boundaries for critical creative action. The BOUNCEBACK work recognised that we may need to define new goals and change the focus of the intended outcome for care. But all three case studies demonstrate that staff (and patients) need supportive goals and frameworks within which they can evaluate the knowledge work of daily practice.

Wise Places need to be cognitive LEARNING spaces: whether learning at the level of individual patients, or learning about the process and impact of systems of care. We need to build the space (protected and prioritised time) and resources (data, expertise) for learning into our new models of generalist practice. Until now, learning (as distinct from service monitoring) has been seen as an 'added extra', often an 'unaffordable luxury' in everyday practice. In our new model of practice, this must change.

I will return to all of these in Chapter 6 when I present a Wise Blueprint for a new model of general practice. But before I do, in the next chapter I first want to look at the system-level factors that may need to change if we are to strengthen Medical Generalism, Now!

REFERENCES

Bryce C et al. (2018). Implementing change in primary care: Lessons from a mixed method evaluation of a frailty initiative. BJGP Open. DOI: 10.3399/bjgpopen18X101421

Dixon-Woods M et al. (2006). Conducting a critical interpretive synthesis of the literature on access to healthcare by vulnerable groups. BMC Medical Research Methodology, 6, p. 35.

Finch TL et al. (2018). Improving the normalisation of complex interventions part 2: Validation of the NoMAD instrument for assessing implementation work based on normalisation process theory. BMC Medical Research Methodology, 18, p. 135.

Fuller C. (2022). Next Steps for Integrating Primary Care: Fuller Stocktake Report. NHS England.

Gulliford M et al. (2002). What does 'access to healthcare' mean? Journal of Health Service Research and Policy, 7, pp. 186–188.

Kovandžić M et al. (2011). Access to primary mental health care for hard to reach groups: From 'silent suffering' to 'making it work. Social Science and Medicine, 72, pp. 763–772.

May CR et al. (n.d.). Normalisation Process Theory. https://normalization-process-theory.northumbria.ac.uk/

Reeve J et al. (2016). Developing, delivering and evaluating primary mental health care: The co-production of a new complex intervention. BMC Health Services Research, 16, p. 470.

Reeve J, Bancroft R. (2014). Generalist solutions to overprescribing: A joint challenge for clinical and academic primary care. Primary Health Care Research & Development, 15(1), pp. 72–79.

Stufflebeam DL. (1973). Evaluation as enlightenment for decision-making. In Worthen BR & Sanders JR. (Eds.), Educational Evaluation: Theory and Practice (pp. 143–147). Worthington, OH: Charles A. Jones Publishing.

CHAPTER 5

Wise systems: The advanced generalist healthcare system

So far, I have recognised the changes needed in professional training and practice, as well as in how we design and run the general practice settings if we want to enable consistent and high-quality advanced generalist care. I now want to take a further step back and consider the wider context in which we work. The priorities and policies of healthcare systems shape every aspect of our work – how we are trained, the contracts and settings we work within, the priorities and resources for healthcare practice, how our work is monitored and evaluated, and the social and societal stories that drive healthcare demand and delivery. In this, the third of my case study chapters, I want to focus on the redesign of health policy and health systems needed to support modern medical generalism and the specialty of whole person medicine. Once again, I will use three case studies to explore the issues – CATALYST, TAILOR and United Generalism. But let me start by briefly describing the policy context in which each of these cases take place – the current status of healthcare policy in the UK.

5.1 SETTING THE SCENE: NEW PUBLIC MANAGEMENT

In this chapter, I consider how the design and delivery of healthcare systems shapes, and ultimately enables or disables, the work of medical generalism.

Knowledge work is the work we do to create understanding (or new knowledge) and then use that knowledge to achieve a goal. Our understanding of many aspects of current healthcare systems (including

DOI: 10.1201/9781003297222-5

defining quality, safety and efficiency) is shaped by the principles of New Public Management (NPM). This approach is so engrained in the culture of the UK health service, the training of healthcare professionals, that it often goes unrecognised and unchallenged. So this is where I start as we think about how we can change.

The NHS was founded over 70 years ago but the systems that underpin its work have adapted and changed over time. The last significant change came around the time I started my career in medicine. This isn't a book about the history of medicine, or medicine management theory, and I would encourage anyone wanting to understand these issues in more depth to explore the work of authors such as Sally Sheard and Ruth McDonald. But I will briefly describe some of the elements that have shaped the knowledge work under discussion here.

In the early decades of the health service, the knowledge work of healthcare practice was defined and controlled by health professionals. The clinician expert defined best care. Opinions of best care were passed on through professional training. Scientific evidence informed discussions, but the doctor was the 'knowledge controller'.

This all changed in the 1980s. As healthcare expanded (both in demand and provision), and costs escalated, the holders of the public purse sought greater control over the design and implementation of healthcare systems. In the interest of greater efficiency, and quality and safety, including the reduction in perceived unacceptable variation in care, we see the introduction of the approach described by Hood (1991) as NPM.

The principles of NPM essentially describe three steps needed for efficient, effective care. Firstly, we should describe 'best care' (evidence-based medicine and the creation of NICE contribute to this). Then, we describe how best care can be delivered – the model of care needed. Thirdly, we implement a system to monitor that care has been correctly delivered and the anticipated outcomes achieved. So, for example, take the case of hypertension and our use of guidelines to optimise care. The NHS has created, and authorised, expert bodies to generate the guidelines – currently, this is the National Institute for Health and Care Excellent (NICE). Convened panels of experts critically examine the (externally produced) scientific evidence to define the criteria for a diagnosis of hypertension. This definition sets the framework, or boundaries, for best diagnostic practice. From an NPM perspective, if a patient is recognised as having blood pressure readings within these boundaries, then best practice describes that they should be diagnosed with hypertension and offered treatment to restore an 'appropriate' blood pressure unless appropriate exceptions exist.

Fred is 50 and has come for a well man's check. His blood pressure is recorded on three separate occasions at a pretty consistent level of 150/90. Fred meets the criteria for a diagnosis of hypertension.

A patient diagnosed with hypertension then enters an evidence-defined pathway of best-practice care to assess the cause of their raised blood pressure and to identify best management. Having implemented a management plan, the system then requires that Fred's blood pressure is reassessed to record that his blood pressure is now back to defined appropriate levels.

Fred underwent a full assessment of cardiovascular risk and was ultimately started on medication to lower his blood pressure. At a review appointment, his blood pressure was now back in target and so the medication was continued with a planned annual review.

Of course, the reality of clinical practice is (or perhaps should be) more complex than this. First and foremost, Fred's priorities and concerns must be factored into this conversation. Shared decision-making (SDM) tools (as discussed in Chapter 3) attempt to ensure that Fred's voice is part of this decision-making process. But SDM tools focus on helping Fred be part of a biomedical decision – to treat his hypertension or not. The diagnosis, for example, has been defined (and so assigned) externally. Of course, Fred and his doctor can agree not to diagnose him with hypertension, but within an NPM system that would be recognised as an 'exception' to 'best practice'. The monitoring systems in today's UK general practice describe it as 'exception reporting'. There is a (strong) implication designed into the healthcare system that this is, at best, not ideal – and potentially wrong.

Managing hypertension seems, at first glance, to be a simple example of how NPM works well. It describes an easily defined problem, with well-described evidence on what to do about it which can be designed into models of care. From a health systems point of view, we can easily measure 'correct' and 'successful' care, and identify care that has not met the standard. In these cases, we can then critically examine the appropriateness of, and reasons for, that exception. There is a nice clear pathway that describes what we should do, how we can do it, and measures if we have achieved success.

This seems like obvious good practice, surely – reducing an individual's risk of developing life-threatening heart disease through 'simple' measures of controlling their blood pressure. There is some benefit to Fred, but an even greater benefit to the wider population. By treating lots of Freds, we can reduce the burden of cardiovascular disease on our communities and our health systems. But even this apparently simple example highlights the complications and limitations of the linear approaches of NPM when we remember we are dealing with people, not just disease states. Ethically, we must recognise Fred as an individual living his daily life, not a means to an end for population health management. But at a systems level, the picture is more complex too. For this, we need to look at the wider evidence base around management of cardiovascular risk.

NPM-driven improvements in the organisation and coordination of healthcare for cardiovascular management has demonstrably contributed to improvements in population health outcomes. Simon Capewell's impact programme (https://impact.ref.ac.uk/casestudies/CaseStudy.aspx?Id=3865) shows that improvements in the medical management of cardiovascular disease account for around 50% of the reduction in cardiovascular deaths (Unal et al. 2004) – a change that is re produced around the world (Bruthans et al. 2014). However, his work also consistently demonstrates that the other 50% reduction is explained by wider public health factors. Improvements in health for populations and individuals has come from improvements in wealth, housing, environmental factors and so on. With growing concern about the burden placed on individuals and health systems by linear healthcare models for managing risk and disease (Chapter 1), do we need to think more creatively about healthcare management? Managing hypertension and cardiovascular risk isn't as straightforward as a condition-focused NPM health system would have us believe.

It is important that we recognise that healthcare is just one (small) factor contributing to improvements in population health. Overreliance on medical management – command and control of disease – has been criticised for contributing to new burdens of healthcare, as well as growing inequalities in health (WHO 1978). But it is not just the 'command and control' goals of healthcare that have been criticised. The delivery of healthcare – and specifically the model of NPM – has been challenged from the outset (Hood 1991; Harrison and Wood 2000). A linear, diagnostic model of healthcare defined by epidemiology and correct diagnosis has been criticised by many for the lack of flexibility to deal with the personal challenges of illness, and the complexity of multimorbidity and comorbidity (see, for example, Tinetti and Fried 2004). Disciplines outside of specialist medicine were particularly vocal against the inflexibility of the medical evidence hierarchy of evidence-based medicine and NPM.

Alternatives to new public management

Management theorists have written extensively on the introduction of NPM, its pros and cons and the implications for current and future public sector management. Harrison and Woods (2000) developed a critique of NPM in healthcare comparing the changes in health systems in the UK and US. They described a political goal behind the introduction of NPM in the 1980s and 1990s – namely to reduce the control of the medical profession in defining the work of healthcare, thus giving greater control back to government over the healthcare budget and expenditure.

The reason I raise that discussion here is to remind us that the way our health system works is a choice based on values and goals. How we define and implement healthcare is not defined by science, or scientific evidence, but by the way we use that science to achieve the goals we want our healthcare systems to meet. Critiques of NPM have proposed that the primary goal behind current healthcare management systems is to keep the control of the boundaries of healthcare in the hands of those who manage the purse strings. Whilst understandable, the unintended consequence of this approach has been to reduce the (perceived) control of healthcare experts to adapt and shape healthcare to the changing needs of the people and populations they work with. NPM builds on management theory developed in industries outside of healthcare. Those settings have now moved on in their thinking. Management theory grounded in the mass production, assembly line practice of 1920s. Ford and Taylorism have moved on to develop new approaches recognising the importance of enabling and optimising the power of human resources to manage ever more complex processes. Is it time for healthcare to follow suit?

NPM has been embedded into UK healthcare systems for more than three decades now. For health professionals and managers working in modern healthcare, it is the 'accepted' model of practice and embedded in the everyday work we do. As I described in the hypertension example, it shapes how we respond to both problems and success – it shapes the culture of our health system. But if we want to respond to the voices calling for culture shift (including Ridge 2021; Fuller 2022; Tinetti and Fried 2004; WHO 1978), we need to take a critical look at the design of the systems in which we work. In this chapter, I want to explore the potential, and opportunities, for using the knowledge work principles I have considered for patient care (Chapter 3), and practice-level design (Chapter 4) to achieve that. I have described how knowledge work can help us change patient and practice-level care, so can it help us change system-level practice?

Once again, I will use three case studies to explore these issues: CATALYST, TAILOR and United Generalism. Each case study builds on the core concepts introduced in earlier chapters and describes the gaps in our current systems that need to be addressed if we are to achieve a system supporting Medical Generalism, Now. Each case study describes how changes to knowledge work, and learning, processes are dependent on system-level changes, but can also be a driver for reform.

I conclude by synthesising the findings from each case study to describe the key system-level inputs needed for medical generalism healthcare reform. The findings in this chapter, along with those preceding, inform the 'manifesto' proposals outlined in Chapter 6 – the new Wise Systems, structures and practice that I argue are needed to deliver healthcare fit for modern needs.

5.2 CATALYST: KNOWLEDGE WORK DRIVERS FOR SYSTEM CHANGE, A WORKFORCE EXAMPLE

Let's start with a people and workforce example of system change that potentially enables whole person, generalist care. I will introduce the example of the CATALYST programme.

CATALYST is a professional development programme, commissioned by NHS England Yorkshire to support new to practice GPs across the region. The programme started with two goals: to address problems with GP recruitment and retention in the area, and to help new to practice GPs build the skills and confidence for the complex reality of the daily practice they were experiencing when they left their vocational training schemes.

Working with local primary care partners, I led the work to design, implement and evaluate this new programme. The design was grounded in the knowledge work principles described in this book – building the skills and confidence to work safely and effectively beyond the boundaries of guidelines and diseases to deliver whole person healthcare at individual consultation and practice levels. I worked with primary care leaders, GPs, practice staff and experts in both education and research using the principles of Transformational Learning Theory (Box 5.1) to describe how we could deliver the programme. As with many recent

BOX 5.1 TRANSFORMATIONAL LEARNING THEORY

Transformational Learning Theory essentially recognises that learners need to experience both the principles or theory of a way of working, and its practical application in context. Both elements are needed to enable the learner to critically reflect on their past understanding of a topic and generate new understanding.

There are three key elements in the use of Transformational Learning Theory in practice: described by Jack Mezirow (Mezirow, 1991) as critical reflection, rational disclosure and centrality of experience. For a learning experience to prompt new understanding for an individual, they need to be actively supported to critically explore and so generate explanations of their new understanding. This needs to actively involve them in open (shared) critical reflection on their own experience of front-line practice. They use the new learning experiences to critically examine and create new understanding.

Transformational Learning Theory is an applied, practical approach to enabling knowledge work in practice.

initiatives, COVID-19 and the lockdown created some unanticipated challenges and indeed opportunities. CATALYST launched in 2021.

Embedded in the CATALYST programme was an evaluation informed by the lessons we learned from implementing the BOUNCEBACK programme (Chapter 4). Our starting point was using Normalisation Process Theory to support a 'trial and learn' approach to building and shaping the new programme. We ought to capture data linked to the outcomes predicted in our impact model (see Figure 5.1 from Dell Olio 2023).

The CATALYST programme recognised four key barriers to generalist knowledge work in context (Permission, Skills, Prioritisation and Performance Management). It aimed to introduce three enablers of practice based on existing education and professional development theory (knowledge work skills training, evidence-informed legitimisation of practice and practical application to everyday problems). The intended (and observed) outcomes were enhanced clinician confidence, skills and job satisfaction.

Enabling knowledge work for practice: What we did

CATALYST essentially aims to support participating GPs to develop skills and confidence in the 4Es of advanced generalist practice – generating, using and critiquing knowledge in context. We use a mixture

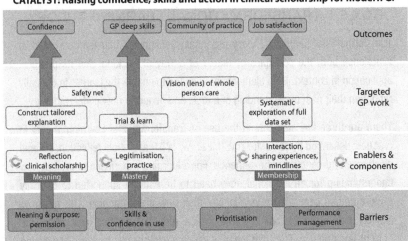

CATALYST: Raising confidence, skills and action in clinical scholarship for modern GP

Figure 5.1   CATALYST impact model.

of theory and applied practice to enable learners to explore, develop understanding, use, and critique the processes described within the 4Es. CATALYST GPs explore a range of data and information sources within the practical examples – research evidence from both healthcare and wider, experiential knowledge from within the group and wider and patient and practice case studies. Tutors stimulate engagement with, and reflection on, the materials to facilitate learning.

Our programme was designed to tackle the four barriers to advanced generalist practice discussed in Chapter 2. To address Permission, we sought to offer our GPs both the understanding of a distinct form of advanced practice, and the evidence that supports its use. We described the building blocks of generalist practice as discussed in Chapter 1, the scientific principles of knowledge work from Chapter 2 including the knowledge of its use in context, and the historical and policy-level calls for a change in culture of practice that have been weaved through this book.

To build skills and confidence in the Professional Action of advanced generalist practice, we used transformational learning principles. In the first 6 months of the course, students focus on clinical scenarios to develop their skills and confidence – challenges such as managing multimorbidity, problematic polypharmacy and persistent physical symptoms. In the next 6 months, they tackle practice-level issues when they are facilitated to undertake a real-world Quality Improvement project. To date, the groups have tackled issues such as improving the care for women experiencing problems with menopausal symptoms, improving the use and recording of paracetamol prescribing and addressing access to the on-call GP. In year 2, CATALYST students look at the wider challenges of lifelong professional practice – becoming leaders of the medical discipline of GP, building and running the multidisciplinary team that is the general practice team and understanding and influencing the wider policy and political agenda that shapes the design of primary care in modern healthcare.

In the first 18 months of running the CATALYST programme, we have had an embedded evaluation designed to describe what is happening, what helps and hinders, and what are the effects of the programme on the learner (Dell Olio 2023). This work is led by Dr Myriam Dell Olio – a lecturer in my research group, whose PhD and doctoral work critically examines everyday epistemology in healthcare settings. As with our BOUNCEBACK work, her evaluation uses action-learning principles where she is embedded in the daily work of the design and delivery of CATALYST, but bringing an external critical gaze to critically understanding that everyday work.

The evaluation demonstrated that CATALYST had multiple impacts: changing the skills and confidence of clinicians in managing everyday complex problems (with implications also for motivation, recruitment and retention); changing practice culture to welcome the expertise of the advanced generalist approach alongside that of specialist medicine; and changing how primary care communities work together in extended communities of practice. The participating GPs valued the reflective knowledge work and interactive learning prompted by CATALYST activities, which led them, in turn, to develop a new understanding of, and confidence in, the skills of advanced practice. By enabling the skills of knowledge work within our cohort of CATALYST GPs, we are delivering on the goals that our funders set us – to improve professional motivation (and so retention), along with enhancing confidence and skills for the everyday work of modern, complex general practice.

But that evaluation is also telling us *how* this happened – *why* CATALYST has achieved its two goals. The evaluation describes three elements of the programme that explain its impact. Firstly, it is changing the GPs sense of professional identity. CATALYST GPs understanding of the role of a new to practice GP has shifted from being defined by what they know (a jack of all trades) to realising it is how they use what they know which offers greatest results to both patients and communities. CATALYST is helping GPs to recognise their expertise as a knowledge worker – not just someone able to apply algorithms repeatedly and efficiently, but a highly skilled professional creating and actioning complex decisions. By recognising and valuing their distinct and valuable advanced generalist skills, CATALYST GPs feel remotivated by the challenges of their daily work. Secondly, is the importance of the transformational learning approach that is enabling GPs to develop, use and learn from these skills in everyday practice. Thirdly, the evaluation highlights the importance of building a Community of Practice within the CATALYST cohort. By having ringfenced, supported (facilitated) cognitive spaces in which to collectively explore the knowledge work of daily practice, GPs gain confidence in the skills and knowledge they create and use; and develop an important and extended 'safety net' for the 'trial and learn' (evaluation) element of their knowledge work.

By enabling knowledge work through the CATALYST programme, we are delivering the culture shift and change in practice that policy makers seek (Ridge 2021; Fuller 2022). But our experience and discussions are also highlighting how healthcare policy will need to change if we are to sustain and scale these shifts, which is what I want to focus on in this chapter – what we're learning from the CATALYST evaluation which helps us understand the policy-level implications for advanced generalist practice.

What we found: Enabling knowledge work

I have described how evaluation work has highlighted three 'active ingredients' in the successful delivery of CATALYST: shifting professional identity, transformational development of knowledge work skills in context and building a community of practice to support ongoing practice and learning. Each has implications for healthcare policy – the systems we build to support and sustain healthcare delivery.

Changing professional identity

CATALYST is working because it is challenging, changing and enhancing people's understanding of what it means to be a GP. It is changing people's perceptions of their professional roles – what their role is (and could be), what skills they need and how they work to do the job. In turn, this is impacting positively on their motivation for the job – with important implications for building and sustain quality healthcare provision.

CATALYST GPs are moving on from the view of a GP as a jack of all trades to instead recognising themselves as highly skilled professionals – 'consultants' in primary care medicine with distinct and valuable skills and expertise; of value not just in the patient consultation but to the running of practice too. CATALYST is supporting GPs to recognise a new vision of advanced professional practice, and with that shift in perception comes a changing sense of motivation for the job and the profession. These changes link to growing confidence in using a distinct skill set that is under-recognised and supported in traditional training and professional development – namely the knowledge work of clinical practice. GPs reveal growing confidence in the mastery of advanced generalist knowledge work, and of an extended professional role.

Some of this is about changing training for professional practice – as discussed in Chapter 3. But it also highlights a need to recognise a different role for the advanced generalist physician: in the healthcare system, and within a primary care, general practice team. We need to rethink the way we understand (and contract) with general practice as organisational units – to motivate and reward the professional autonomy needed for complex, advanced practice (the knowledge work of practice). We need to update models of practice away from the linear, transactional focus of NPM models to newer management systems that provide the frameworks for safe but effective complex working.

By foregrounding the knowledge work of professional practice in the CATALYST programme, we have changed understanding and engagement of professionals with primary care practice. CATALYST GPs are motivated to want to continue in practice and roll out wider changes. Foregrounding knowledge work is acting as a driver for systems change.

Prioritising shared creative spaces for transformational learning

The second successful element of CATALYST has been in creating spaces. CATALYST created a protected space for shared knowledge work that is in turn enabling and supporting the wider application of knowledge work in everyday practice. But what do we mean by 'space' – what is an effective space?

CATALYST GPs come out of practice for 2 days a month to take part in the programme. Some people have questioned whether the benefit of CATALYST is simply giving people a regular break from the challenges of front-line practice. CATALYST GPs meet regularly with a group of people, and get to know each other through the programme. So is this what I mean by space – a sociable time out to relax?

Well, no. The evaluation of CATALYST demonstrates that those spaces need to cognitive spaces designed to specifically support transformational learning. They need to support, and reinforce, the understanding and practice of advanced professional skills that I have discussed. To do that, they need to be critical, creative learning spaces – spaces for knowledge work. As will also be reflected in my next case study (TAILOR), those spaces also need to be resourced. Protected time is about prioritising and legitimising this work – recognising it as an integral part of everyday professional practice. It is no bolt-on, nice to do if you have time, for your own personal good (potentially to be done in your own time). Rather, it is an integral part of everyday professional practice and, therefore, needs to be designed into our workplaces and spaces.

CATALYST is also demonstrating that it is insufficient to just put people into a cognitive space and expect them to work it out for themselves. Advanced knowledge work is a 'team sport'. To take that further, let me return to the scientific principles that underpin this work which I discussed in Chapter 2. My academic role involves me in knowledge work every day. My role expects, and requires, me to work with others in that task. I would not, for example, be funded to do a piece of research that I hadn't developed and discussed with other researchers as well as experts from outside of research (patients, clinicians and so on). My working week is designed to support and enable the conversations necessary to support the critical, creative knowledge work processes needed to deliver robust and impactful research. What CATALYST highlights is how and why we need to design that into clinical knowledge work spaces too.

Again, this requires a culture shift for health systems. They currently perceive that knowledge work takes place outside of the clinical setting (in NICE for example). Healthcare settings are designed for transactional delivery of the units of care described by the external knowledge work. CATALYST highlights why and how that needs to change. To introduce knowledge work into everyday practice, and so achieve the benefits of Medical Generalism now, we need to change the vision and design of the healthcare system. This includes changing the systems vision of the roles of the professionals working within healthcare. We also need to change the way that work is organised: the description and delegation of roles within and across teams, and the organisation of the 'working week'. I will return to this in Chapter 6.

Permission for learning: A learning organisation

CATALYST is describing a potential system-level shift in our understanding of professional identity and of the critical creatives (knowledge work) activities needed within the workspace. Both elements are necessary to enable clinicians, and so the healthcare systems they work for, deal with complexity and the inevitable 'messiness' of everyday person-centred practice. But one of the concerns that led to the introduction of our current NPM models of 'transactional' healthcare was a stated desire to reduce unacceptable variations in care. Giving healthcare professionals autonomy (or too much autonomy) in decisions about healthcare potentially allows too much scope for 'bad practice'. We had data on the actions of healthcare systems which showed differences in how healthcare was working in different places. The proposed solution for this 'unacceptable variation' was to seek to standardise the work of the healthcare community.

Returning to the example of Fred and the management of his blood pressure, let's look at it from the healthcare system perspective. Fred's clinical record shows that his blood pressure is in the hypertensive range but that he hasn't been started on a blood pressure medication. How can the system tell whether Fred has had poor condition-specific/specialist care or excellent advanced generalist care? It is not possible to tell from routine NHS data whether Fred's care was sub-standard – his blood pressure was missed, or the clinician wasn't up to date with the guidelines – or a decision based on best advanced generalist practice using a 4E conversation with Fred. What if Fred then goes on to have a stroke: how do we distinguish between poor specialist clinical care, and good generalist care where Fred was unlucky? We can 'exception report' Fred from guideline care – to send a message to the healthcare system that standard care wasn't right for him. But this doesn't say anything about whether the care he received instead was good or not. It is an example of the Performance Monitoring barrier discussed in Chapter 1: at best, clinicians receive no feedback on their practice; at worst, they are criticised for not following guideline care.

Of course there are millions of Freds (and Fredas) in our community. The healthcare system is trying to monitor best care from a whole population perspective. It doesn't have the capacity to look at each individual case. From this perspective, we can see the appeal of an NPM system which sets targets, designs delivery processes and checks compliance. It perhaps feels like the lowest risk, and most scalable option.

Yet, our experience of today's healthcare systems (whether as patients or clinicians) is now demonstrating the limitations of this approach. In my everyday clinical practice, I see relatively few Freds; but many more people like Elsie (see Chapter 3) – people living with multiple long-term conditions, which interconnect and interact, making the decisions much more complex. As I have discussed throughout this book, whole person healthcare is messy, non-linear, complex and changeable. Therefore, we need to build capacity into our healthcare systems to deal with this inevitable uncertainty and constant change. The third element that CATALYST has flagged is the need to enable and support LEARNING as integral to everyday practice.

But we need to be clear what learning is, and isn't, in this context. Generalist Learning is not about audit – have you done what you were supposed to do and corrected any elements that you missed. Learning is not about acquiring knowledge – updating on the latest guidelines. Instead, learning is about creating, using and critiquing knowledge in context. This learning work needs to be designed into systems – in the way we describe roles and allocate resources including time. CATALYST highlights that it must also be designed into the way we performance manage our healthcare systems: developing new ways to monitor and maintain good practice beyond just the delivery of guideline-concordant care.

In conclusion

Knowledge work is part of the solution to the culture and system changes needed to deliver whole-person-centred healthcare; in particular through championing the greatest resource in the NHS – its workforce. By creating an enabled and motivated workforce, we may start to deliver the positive change and culture shift (Ridge 2021; Fuller 2022) that is urgently needed in our healthcare systems.

5.3 TAILOR: KNOWLEDGE WORK DRIVERS FOR SYSTEM CHANGE, A WORKPLACE EXAMPLE

In my second case study, I want to shift the focus away from the professionals delivering healthcare to consider instead the context in which they meet and work. I have already explored how the goals of healthcare (to command and control of disease, or optimise whole person health for daily living) shape everyday clinical practice and decision making. Those goals also shape how we create the healthcare settings in which people work. If we understand the purpose of healthcare to optimise disease management, for example, this will shape how we design access to healthcare. Access systems will focus on assessing and addressing disease risk. This perspective will shape the resources we allocate to healthcare (data, work allocation and prioritisation, governance and monitoring, and many more). These elements are all identified as potential barriers to advanced generalist practice by front-line clinicians (see Chapter 2).

Therefore, if we want to enable generalist care, we need to address those barriers by changing the contexts in which generalist practitioners work. So what does a generalist healthcare workplace need and what are the specific implications for healthcare systems arising from that?

I will explore these questions by thinking about a key challenge facing today's healthcare patients, professionals, practices and systems – the issue of problematic polypharmacy. In summer 2021, the Chief Pharmaceutical Officer for England published a report in Overprescribing in the NHS. His report highlighted that in 2019, approximately 27 million people in England were taking at least one medicine regularly (more than half the population), 15% of patients were taking five or more medicines a day and 7% were on eight or more. Janet Krska's research has shown that of those people taking five or more medicines a day, 40% report feeling burdened by their medicines (Krska et al. 2018). Burden isn't caused just by side effects, but the whole impact of using medicines on daily living. Medicines must be ordered, collected, organised and taken at the right time in the right way. This can mean changing other daily activities and routines so this can happen. There are follow-up and monitoring activities to be done and appointments to be kept. People may have effects from their medicines that need to be accommodated. All of this adds to the burden of treatment and illness that I discussed in Chapter 1. Perhaps the most hidden aspect is the effect on people's sense of self and identity – their creative capacity (Chapter 1). For some people, having to take medicines every day leaves them feeling 'not the same as I was', or 'no longer healthy' – creating significant identity work to do. In other cases, medicines become seen as 'the thing that is keeping me alive' (whether that is medically 'accurate' or not); adding to a burden of health anxiety, and significantly shaping how people live their daily lives (Reeve and Cooper 2014).

Some medicines are, indeed, key to 'keeping people alive', having a significant positive effect on their health for daily living and quality of life. Take the example of Bill, who lives with Parkinson's disease. Without l dopa, he would spend much of his life 'locked in' to a body unable to manage its neurological function unaided. But for Fred on his antihypertensives, the situation is different. These medicines are not keeping him alive and functioning *today* – they are addressing a longer-term risk. For many individuals, the personal absolute benefit of antihypertensives is small – the greatest benefit is a societal one with potentially significant reduction in population-level risk and disease status. If Fred is not feeling burdened by his medication, and values the risk reduction it offers to him personally, then continuing the medicines is appropriate. But if the perceived burden to Fred outweighs the potential benefit, then continuing the medication becomes problematic. If we were to continue antihypertensives in this situation, we would effectively be using Fred as a means to an end – treating him for the population (and health system's) benefit – which is, of course, ethically unacceptable.

Antihypertensives are one of the most commonly prescribed medicines in UK healthcare. We have well-described pathways of care supporting the decision to start medication and to review whether it is working – models linked to the NPM approach I discussed at the beginning of this chapter. Hypertension management is often viewed at an organisational level as a relatively straightforward task – that can be clearly described and monitored, and so also delegated to appropriately trained staff in the team, but not usually needing medical input. Yet, my discussion of Fred flags up the potential for this to be more complex than appears at first glance. This complexity is compounded if Fred is one of the 15% of people taking multiple medicines every day. We need to consider the additional challenges of dealing with polypharmacy – the use of multiple medicines for one individual on a long-term basis.

The Kings Fund wrote a report on this issue in 2013. Their report highlighted the potential benefits of using multiple medicines on quality and longevity of life, but also the potential challenges and harms in terms of burden and adverse effects. That report proposed that we need to recognise, and distinguish between, so-called appropriate polypharmacy and problematic polypharmacy (see Box 5.2). They also

---

BOX 5.2 KINGS FUND (2013) DEFINITIONS OF POLYPHARMACY

'Appropriate polypharmacy is defined as prescribing for an individual for complex conditions or for multiple conditions in circumstances where medicines use has been optimised and where the medicines are prescribed according to best evidence'.

'Problematic polypharmacy is defined as the prescribing of multiple medications inappropriately, or where the intended benefit of the medication is not realised'.

In deciding whether polypharmacy is appropriate (optimised) or problematic (intended benefit is not realised), 'the patient perspective on medication-taking needs to be determined and recorded. Compromises may often need to be reached between the view of the prescriber in delivering interventions intended to improve outcome, and the choice made by the patient, based on the demands of the medication regimen'.

described that when polypharmacy becomes a problem, we will need to actively recognise that decision making will need to include compromise in our decision making about if and when to use medicines. Denford et al. (2014) have described this as the need for 'mutually agreed tailoring' of decisions about medicine use through discussion and agreement between clinician and patient.

Compromise and mutually agreed tailoring of decisions are not clearly designed into the NPM systems described at the beginning of this chapter. We can opt people out of routine, guideline described care (exception reporting) but systems are not designed to proactively offer and support mutually tailored care. As discussed, my research has highlighted the system-level barriers to tailored care including Permission, Prioritisation and Performance Management. So what elements are needed in a new system of care that supports tailored prescribing? Answering this question was the focus of the TAILOR project.

Introducing TAILOR

In 2019, the National Institute for Health Research invited proposals to undertake a review of the evidence of the safety and effectiveness of deprescribing – or stopping medication – especially in older people living with multiple long-term conditions and experiencing medication burden. Reading between the lines, the funders were hoping that researchers could systemically pool all the evidence on describing to generate a new evidence-based summary that would tell clinicians how best to stop which medicines, in which patients and with what anticipated effect. In other words, they were asking: Could the evidence be used to produce new (linear) pathways describing how to stop medicines to use alongside the existing pathways that tell us when to start medicines?

You won't be surprised that our research team challenged these assumptions – for all the reasons I have been outlining in this book so far. However, we did want to add an evidence-informed critical voice to the wider discussions on how to tackle problematic polypharmacy highlighted, for example, in the Ridge review. So having secured the funding, we set about systematically reviewing the literature to understand the system-level changes needed to tackle the growing phenomenon of problematic polypharmacy. Our proposal was that we need to introduce system-level changes to support *tailored* deprescribing in people at risk of, or experiencing, problematic polypharmacy. (Our review therefore focused on older people over 50 years of age, taking five or more medicines a day, and with three or more long-term conditions.) We sought to answer two questions: Is it safe and acceptable to discontinue medicines in this patient group? How, for whom and in what contexts can safe and effective tailoring of clinical decisions related to medication use work to produce the desired outcomes?

Should we stop long-term medicines?

Our first question considered whether it was safe, effective and acceptable to stop medicines in this patient group. In other words, should we even consider tailoring medicines – working beyond guidelines describing medication to be used for different conditions, and building in 'compromise' shaped by individual needs and contexts. This first stage of our work looked to address the barriers of Permission and Performance Management described in Chapter 1.

The full details of how we did this work, and our findings, are in the final report available in the NIHR library (Reeve et al. 2022). Essentially, we created a map of the field of research evidence out there and used that to look in detail at the issues of safety, acceptability and effectiveness of tailored deprescribing. The research studies included in our review covered a whole range of clinical situations – stopping different types of medicines, in different clinical scenarios, and using different clinical tools to help. The research map is very messy. Our approach was to look for patterns in the data – areas where, despite the diversity, there seemed to be clear messages of positive effect (green flags) or negative (red flags).

From many months of work, we were able to draw some clear conclusions from that work. Firstly, the evidence demonstrates that deprescribing is potentially safe, effective and acceptable if done in a structured way. Studies consistently revealed more benefit than harm in situations where the clinicians had used a structured tool or approach to support and describe their approach. There was no consistent data or evidence to demonstrate that any one clinical tool was better than another. Some studies used recognised tools such as Beers, STOPP/START and TRIM; others used a framework such as Reeve et al.'s (2017) 7 steps for deprescribing. Both approaches were acceptable, and more effective, than studies which did not use (or report) a structured clinical approach that had been applied in managing medicines.

Secondly, there is a lot of unexplained variation in the data – as would be expected for a complex situation – meaning that using tailored deprescribing to manage problematic polypharmacy is not a simple (linear) process generating a defined outcome. The review flagged the need to recognise tailored care within the interpretive knowledge work framework that I have described for advanced generalist care, rather than the hypothetico-deductive pathway of guideline-focused specialist care. This led us to our second research question: The need to understand how this can be safely done and what elements do we need in healthcare systems to support this?

What do we need in place to enable tailored medication use?

We answered this second question, again, with an analysis of the published evidence on medicines use. This time we used a research method that allows us to dig into the data within the published research to understand what is happening and how things work (or don't). This method is known as a realist review and, again, full details of how we did this work are in the final report. This piece of work involved us in another detailed review and synthesis of a large body of research over many months to critically examine the processes and contexts that shape prescribing practice. We quickly realised our preliminary findings were echoing the observations raised in the reports from both the Kings Fund and Ridge. The research evidence also highlighted that to understand and potentially change deprescribing, we needed to critically examine and understand organisational and system-level and cultural factors, professional practice, and patient-level factors. Our methodological approach also allowed us to look at how each level impacted the other.

The realist review method enables the research team to generate a set of evidence-based statements – in this case, about how deprescribing happens. Our review identified a number of factors that impact prescribing work. These are the themes that appeared consistently throughout the evidence and so can be recognised as key drivers for practice. The themes we highlighted included organisation and system-level factors, professional behaviours, patient factors, continuity of care and trust, SDM, multidisciplinary collaboration and monitoring and learning. I'll describe a few examples of what we saw in these themes to help illustrate.

Based on consistent data across the body of research, we were able to state that the literature tells us:

When healthcare providers feel like they cannot make justifiable decisions that are supported by guidelines they may be reluctant to make changes to medications because they are afraid of negative consequences.

(CMOC2, Organisation & System-level theme)

When patients view medicines as prolonging their lives they may be reluctant to stop taking them because they view deprescribing as a sign that they aren't worth keeping alive anymore.

(CMOC16, Patient factors theme)

When healthcare professionals know that they will be able to follow-up a patient, they are more likely to try deprescribing, because they are reassured they will be able to manage potential harms.

(CMOC27, Trust theme)

When healthcare professionals can draw on the skills and expertise of colleagues they feel more confident in making prescription changes because they feel re-assured that they are making safe and optimal prescribing decisions.

(CMOC32, Multidisciplinary collaboration theme)

These are just a few examples from the 34 statements that we produced. The full list is available in the TAILOR report (Reeve et al. 2022). To clinicians reading this book, these statements may seem obvious – just common sense. The difference with the realist method is that these are now evidence-based statements, supported by a consistent literature. Therefore, we now have an evidence-base for our professionally recognised 'common sense' understanding of practice, and so a base from which to potentially challenge and change existing practice.

Through the realist review method, we were able to synthesise the 34 statements that we produced to describe an overarching model of what is needed to support tailored use of medicines or deprescribing. We described this as the DExTruS Framework (see Figure 5.2).

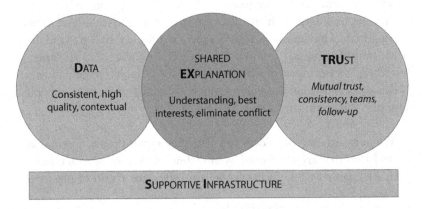

Figure 5.2 The DExTruS framework. (From Reeve et al. 2022.)

DExTruS described four key elements needed to support tailored use of medication: Data, shared Explanations, TRUst, and Supportive infrastructure.

All relate to the knowledge work of prescribing practice, and there are implications for practice and system-level design in all four. I'll start by describing each of the four components and then consider the implications for workplace and system-level redesign to support the knowledge work of tailored prescribing.

Describing DExTrus

Complex tailored decision making needs Data. The NHS is awash with data. What our review demonstrated was that this data needs to be high quality, consistently available and, crucially, that it includes contextual data. Data is needed to support the Exploration necessary to generate mutually agreed tailoring of medicines use. In my account of the Complex Needs work in Chapter 4, I recognised that this information was missing in the records we kept for a group of patients potentially highly vulnerable to problematic polypharmacy. In my clinical experience, contextual data is hard to record well and keep up to date. Traditionally, it is the information that is stored in the head of the clinician who knows this patient well, potentially over a long period of time. TAILOR highlighted that we need to find ways to be better at getting this data out of the heads of clinicians and into the way we design places and systems of healthcare. I'll return to this in Chapter 6.

Tailoring of medicines relies on establishing shared understanding of the goals, potential benefit and harm of medicines, enabling appropriate compromise between biomedical and biographical outcomes. This depends on the creation and use of Shared Explanation – the third E of advanced generalist practice. I've already considered the clinical work needed for this. DExTruS flags the workplace and system changes needed too – data, supportive infrastructure and systems that enable and enhance trust.

The third element is Trust. Denford and colleagues' description of the need for *mutually agreed* tailoring, and the Kings Fund call for *compromise*, both flagged trust as a potential key issue. Of course, trust is recognised as a core value in healthcare (General Medical Council n.d.) and one of the strongest predictors of patient reported trust is that they recognise their problem as being taken seriously, understood, explained and addressed (Croker 2013). What DExTruS added to those accounts was a recognition that building trust needs clear explanations and expectations, consistency across teams and the opportunity for follow-up and continuity of learning.

Two workplace and system-level factors are revealed here. Firstly, the importance of consistency across teams – including the extended teams of practitioners working in primary and secondary care. The review repeatedly highlighted the challenges faced by patients who were told one thing by one clinician and a different story elsewhere. A hospital consultant might tell someone they will be on this medication for the rest of their life. If a primary care generalist clinician later starts a discussion about the utility of this medicine, what the patient hears is (potentially) 'you are reaching the end of your life so it's not worth giving you this medicine any more'. Of course, different clinicians in different contexts may have different perspectives on the usefulness of a medicine. Consistency isn't the same as expecting everyone to say the same thing. But consistency, and trust, does require that each member of the extended team has access to the explanation that other team members have offered to a patient. This highlights the second issue and takes us back to the importance of data – we need consistent access to 'contextual' data which includes what has been explained to the patient before *and why*. TAILOR flags the importance of consistently discussing the whole person implications of using medicines in every discussion we have with patients – certainly when we're discussing medicines that will be taken long term. This is perhaps the thinking behind the Health Education England (2021) Future Doctor report which called for every doctor to be trained in generalist skills. It doesn't mean that every clinician has to undertake a detailed generalist assessment of every patient they see; but it does remind us that all clinical decisions should be mindful of a whole person perspective, a consideration that is ideally recorded and shared in clinical records.

The fourth component of DExTruS is a recognition of the need for a Supportive infrastructure. Elements specifically recognised by the review included policy and incentive structures, clarity of professional roles, recognition of professional parity between generalist and specialist clinicians within extended multidisciplinary teams, building skills and confidence in clinical teams and continuity of care. The review highlighted that system-level changes are needed to enable these to happen.

Implications of TAILOR: Systems design

The TAILOR review provides further evidence-based support for the workforce level changes described at the start of this chapter. We need to review and revise the training and ongoing professional support for clinicians delivering advanced generalist care. But TAILOR also provides evidence for the workplace changes needed too. Specifically, it flags the need to look at TEAMS, LEARNING and DATA.

Digital reform within the NHS is a current priority. The primary focus at the moment is on improving efficiency of healthcare systems and seeking to deliver more care at a faster speed. My concern is that we are trying to do more of the same, quicker. Instead we need to recognise the opportunity for digital technology to support new ways of working – including advanced generalist practice. There is a key opportunity to consider how do we collect and share the right data – including contextual data – across teams, and keep it updated. Perhaps also to consider how we use technology to move unnecessary data out of the way, to avoid important contextual data being crowded out, for example, by service data. I will return to this in Chapter 6.

Team working in the NHS isn't new, although it is changing – and rapidly. Much of the change is being driven by necessity – the need to fill immediate gaps in workforce rotas is a key driver for current decision making, rather than a longer-term consideration of sustained and sustainable care. Our current approach to managing the workforce crisis is, perhaps, similar to the way we are dealing with escalating patient numbers. In both cases, all our attention is on finding immediate 'solutions', or at least quick fixes. We haven't the time or headspace to take a step back and consider why and how the problems have arisen. To use a public health analogy, we are so busy pulling people out of the river, we don't have time to go upstream and consider why they are all falling in. So we aim to recruit more people to build our capacity to do more of the same (rescuing people from the river or problematic polypharmacy); but without considering whether we could work differently upstream to reduce the number of people entering the river (through changing the way we prescribe). We welcome new colleagues into the team, including pharmacists and nurse prescribers. But we haven't spent time working with them, thinking with them, about defining the distinct yet complementary roles that each can provide to this complex work. As the workload grows, we haven't the headspace for those conversations and, instead, we (once again) revert to applying guideline (protocol)-defined models of care to patients – using as many people as possible to keep pulling people out of the river.

TAILOR highlighted the importance of developing tailored Explanations of the use of medicines if we want to implement an upstream approach to managing problematic polypharmacy. Creating explanations uses the knowledge work skills of advanced generalist practice. Implementing tailored prescribing requires that we know where these knowledge work skills sit within the multidisciplinary teams responsible for medicines management. Not every prescriber will have those skills; and not every professional with those skills will be a prescriber. As we welcome an expanding diversity of health professionals into UK general practice at the moment, the TAILOR review reminds us that tailored prescribing will require clear statement of roles and responsibilities across those teams in order to support SDM across a community of practice. This is crucial so that both patients and clinicians can work to generate and maintain Trust in the tailored understanding and management of medicines.

In conclusion

Ridge concluded his review of overprescribing by stating that we need to change our systems and culture in the NHS related to medicines. He called for greater use of personalised decision making; alternatives to medicines for managing health problems; and better recording, sharing and reviewing of medicine-related decision making. All of these will require redesign of practice and policy to enable advanced generalist care; with greater use of the role of 'Generalist Gatekeeper or Guru' (Chapter 3), as well as the system changes described by TAILOR. Problematic polypharmacy is one of the biggest challenges facing the NHS, and indeed Western healthcare systems. My work suggests this problem also offers a powerful opportunity to enable healthcare redesign for advanced generalist care. By tackling problematic polypharmacy using an advanced generalist approach, we can drive wider healthcare reform with wide potential for benefit.

5.4   UNITED GENERALISM: A POLICY EXAMPLE

So far, I have discussed system-level changes needed to support new workforce and workplace design for advanced generalist care. Taking a further step back, I now turn to consider the whole system policy drivers that shape actions and so will also need to change. We need to look again at the goals of healthcare.

In my 25 years' experience of working in primary care, people have most commonly told me that general practice is a 'practical' discipline. It works to get on with the job at hand, to deal with the issues presenting at the door. The goal of care has been defined as doing the job that the patient brings through the door. This understanding of the GP role fits closely with the view of the generalist as a 'jack of all trades'.

In my professional experience, there has been a tendency to avoid, or even reject, wider discussions about the goals of healthcare as 'too academic'. The job is just to get the work done. As one colleague described it, 'General practice has always been good at describing how to do the job, but not necessarily at describing why we do it'.

As primary care now struggles to deal with the 30 million or more consultations with general practice taking place every month in England, I am beginning to see people turn their attention back to the questions of what are we doing, and why. Questions that previously have been considered 'too academic' are now being recognised as very practical questions about what do we need to prioritise, continue and protect in general practice – and also what do we need to consider stopping doing. It is to this broader question about the goals of care that I now return in this final case example and my consideration of the idea of United Generalism.

In the opening chapter, I proposed that a generalist view recognises healthcare as a social commodity intended to help people live their lives. Health is not the primary goal of healthcare; but enabling health as a resource needed for daily living is. The goals of healthcare therefore focus on the outputs of enabled citizens and communities – the individual and social capital that human populations need to survive and thrive.

However, I have also argued that much of the current focus in healthcare is on managing (or 'controlling') disease. We design systems to identify and intervene in disease and, in turn, to monitor the impact of our intervention. Reducing the prevalence and impact of disease is seen as a measure of improving health. Disease status is measured and monitored in an NPM healthcare system. Quality care has become defined as care that we can readily manage and measure, rather than what is necessarily the best care. So I have also explored the unintended consequences of this approach in creating burden for patients, clinicians and health systems alike. With growing prevalence of overmedicalisation, burden of treatment and undertreatment of conditions not readily described by biomedical pathways, international voices have started to question and indeed challenge, a biomedical definition of best care (Tinetti and Fried 2004; WHO 1978). These narratives have led me, and others, to question whether we need to reconsider the goals of healthcare; and so re-define the framework of best practice that guides how we design, resource, deliver and evaluate healthcare.

This issue was debated in an editorial written by Steven Lewis in 2013. He started by recognising that whilst healthcare systems treat 'parts', people break down (or get ill) in 'wholes' (Lewis 2013). His writing considered how can we better organise a healthcare system around the person who is ill, rather than the illness(es) that they have. In doing so, he took a critical look at generalist healthcare.

Lewis described a (potential) need for more generalist healthcare, but his work offered a new look in recognising two emerging 'faces' of generalism. Firstly, he described the principles of what is now commonly referred to as integrated care. Here, whole person healthcare is understood as the need to more effectively and efficiently integrate the multiple facets of specialist care which manage the distinct 'parts' in the 'whole' person. Integrated care describes the ideas that lie behind the current wave of NHS reform.

But Lewis recognised a second face of generalism – the principles described in my work, and presented in this book. He described it as

> a more revolutionary face of generalism – one that challenges the search-and-destroy paradigm of modern scientific medicine. ...a restrained generalism grounded in person-centred care may appear quaint and unambitious, a vegan's conceit in a world of carnivores. But it is relevant to the widespread failures of the here and now, and whether and how it takes hold matters a great deal.
>
> (Lewis 2013)

Of course, I welcomed Lewis's recognition of my ideas and endorsement of the work I was trying to do. I also found his suggestion of two faces really useful – because it highlighted that we need *both*. His writing led me to consider whether these were the two faces of the ancient Roman god of Janus – the god of beginnings, transitions and endings. Perhaps these two faces of generalism describe the past (integration of specialist care) moving into a new future (advanced generalist care). But as both a practising clinician caring for people living with acute and chronic disease, and a patient myself living with a long-term condition, I wanted to have both improved, integrated delivery of specialist-derived healthcare *and* the whole person derived understanding of healthcare that I understand as advanced generalist care. Our healthcare system needs both.

These thoughts led Professor Richard Byng and I to propose a new 'united model of generalism'. We described a unified view that recognises the value and need for both 'coordinated specialist' and 'interpretive advanced generalist' care in an extended vision of an integrated healthcare system (Reeve and Byng 2017).

Our United Generalism model recognised two axes of healthcare delivery (Figure 5.3). One describes the professional knowledge work needed to

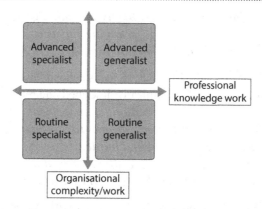

Figure 5.3 United generalism.

deliver healthcare: ranging from specialist to generalist. The other describes the organisational work needed to deliver that care: ranging from routine to advanced. Together, these axes create a two by two matrix re-defining the knowledge work of our extended view of integrated healthcare.

The work needed to care for a patient in each quadrant is different (Figure 5.4):

- ADVANCED SPECIALIST CARE: This is the technically advanced, coordinated care to meet a defined disease state) need – usually needing advanced equipment and resources only found in the hospital setting
  - *Examples include severe trauma care, managing an acute myocardial infarction or stroke and cancer care.*

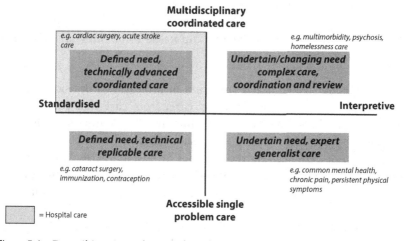

Figure 5.4 Describing 4 quadrants of work in united generalism.

- *Knowledge work involves highly specialist generation of data for decision making (e.g., scanning, invasive care) supporting hypothetico-deductive decision making.*

- ROUTINE SPECIALIST CARE: Delivers defined, disease or condition-focused care, that can be technically described and replicated.
  - *Examples include vaccination, management of acute minor illness and uncomplicated chronic disease management where no concerns about individual burden.*
  - *Knowledge work involves readily managed data collection and interpretation, potentially algorithm-based care.*

- ROUTINE GENERALIST CARE: Deals with uncertain or changing healthcare needs requiring expert generalist (inductive) interpretation and care but which can be managed by staff with 'basic' generalist skills.
  - *Examples may include mild-moderate distress (e.g., described in BOUNCEBACK), chronic pain and persistent physical symptoms at the low-moderate end of spectrum.*
  - *Knowledge work involves inductive data collection to generate an explanation and management plan implemented with the individual patient where care is effective, supportive.*

- ADVANCED GENERALIST CARE: Involves dealing with uncertain or changing healthcare need where complexity adds to the risk of both illness and treatment burden, meaning that healthcare requires coordination and ongoing review.
  - *Examples include severe multimorbidity and frailty care, psychosis care and homelessness care.*
  - *The knowledge work here includes the 4Es supported by DExTruS system models. Care needs to be integrated across a multidisciplinary team.*

Our account recognised a spectrum of professional decision making from 'standardised' to 'interpretive' care: from care that could be fitted to a hypothetico-deductive guideline, to care needing an inductive, interpretive approach. The model also highlighted the relatively small proportion of care needing the facilities of hospital care. Although our intention wasn't primarily to argue for further resources in primary care, it does point to a potential to redesign healthcare spaces (and policy) to support this approach.

My intention in using United Generalism as a case study here is to highlight two major policy shifts needed to enable advanced generalist practice. Firstly, it creates a new additional focus for healthcare from considering the *management* of a condition, to the *work* needed to manage that problem. This creates a new prioritisation (Etz et al. 2021 – see Chapter 2) role for health systems. To deliver whole person care, we need to know more than what conditions a person is living with. We also need to know if that person is at further risk of health and healthcare-related disruption to daily living. In other words, we need to know if the individual needs access to the distinct skills of advance generalist practice. An extended vision of integrated care needs to recognise the 'speciality' (distinct unit of healthcare practice) that is advanced generalist care.

This leads to my second observation – that the extended vision of integrated healthcare described by United Generalism requires us to rethink how we prioritise healthcare resources. A growing proportion of the work of general practice takes place in the Advanced Generalist quadrant, yet the resources and management of are focused on the Routine specialist quadrant. Primary care contracts and performance management systems focus on the bottom-left quadrant, meaning the money flows to that work. Yet, patients experience problems in the top-right quadrant, and clinicians are left trying to manage a growing volume of work in this sector without adequate resource.

Professor Byng and I proposed the need for some consensus work to describe what conditions go in which quadrant. This would enable analysis of the epidemiological burden, and so resource needed, in each quarter. As I look to implement the ideas from Medical Generalism, Now! I hope we can do this work through some on-the-ground knowledge work to redesign general practice – as I will discuss in more Chapter 6.

5.5 IMPLICATIONS FOR MEDICAL GENERALISM, NOW!

The case studies in this chapter have highlighted the system-level changes needed to enable the delivery of advanced Medical Generalism, Now.

I described the need to build into our systems of healthcare: support for knowledge work (including professional training, resources for practice and cognitive spaces for learning), re-prioritisation of need and allocation of resources and clarification and redefinition of team and individual roles within them.

The potential impact of those changes includes enhancing professional capacity and satisfaction, reducing patient burden and de-escalation of demand on healthcare systems. Certainly, we need to shift the direction of current healthcare away from metrics which show we are delivering 1 million GP consultations a day in England, but leaving 40% of GPs planning to quit the profession in the next 5 years (RCGP 2022). I led work in the UK to establish the WiseGP programme: offering a new vision of general practice and the role of the GP as a skilled knowledge worker providing person-centred care in the community context (www.wisegp.co.uk). But a new vision isn't enough, we also need to change practice and policy – hence Medical Generalism, Now!

My intention here is not to describe a simple 'alternative' model of practice: to replace one problematic model with another which would no doubt be equally problematic. Instead, I seek to recognise that current care *systems* cannot do the job. As we described in work we published a few years ago on transforming care for people living with multimorbidity: 'Trying harder will not work, changing systems of care will' (Reeve et al. 2013).

In this chapter, I sought to outline some of the changes to support advanced generalist practice recognised within the case studies described. In the next chapter, I turn to consider what that might look like as a model of general practice on the ground.

REFERENCES

Bruthans J et al. (2014). Explaining the decline in coronary heart disease mortality in the Czech Republic between 1985 and 2007. European Journal of Preventative Cardiology, 21, pp. 829–839.

Croker JE et al. (2013). Factors affecting patients' trust in GPs: Evidence from the English national GP patient survey. BMJ Open, 3, p. e002762.

Dell Olio M. (2023). Evaluation of the CATALYST programme, *in preparation*.

Denford S et al. (2014). Individualisation of drug treatments for patients living with long term conditions: A review of concepts. BMJ Open, 4, p. e004172.

Etz R, Miller W, Stange K. (2021). Simple rules that guide generalist and specialist care. Family Medicine, 53(8), pp. 697–699.

Fuller C. (2022). Next steps for integrating primary care: Fuller Stocktake Report. NHS England.

General Medical Council. (n.d.). Good Medical Practice Domain 4 – maintaining trust. www.gmc-uk.org/ethical-guidance/ethical-guidance-for-doctors/good-medical-practice/domain-4---maintaining-trust

Harrison S, Wood B. (2000). Scientific-bureaucratic medicine and UK health policy. Political Studies Review, 17, pp. 25–42.

Health Education England. (2021). The Future Doctor Report. London: Health Education England.

Hood C. (1991). A public management for all seasons? Public Administration, 69, pp. 3–19.

Kings Fund. (2013). Polypharmacy and Medicines Optimisation. London: Kings Fund.

Krska J, Katusiime B, Corlett S. (2018). Patient experiences of the burden of medicines for long term conditions and factors affecting burden: A cross-sectional study. Health and Social Care in the Community, 26, pp. 946–959.

Lewis S. (2013). The two faces of generalism. Journal of Health Services Policy and Research, 19, pp. 1–2.

Mezirow J. (1991). Transformative Dimensions of Adult Learning. Oxford, Jossey-Bass Ltd.

Reeve J et al. (2013). Generalist solutions to complex problems: Generating practice-based evidence – the example of managing multi-morbidity. BMC Primary Care, 14, p. 112.

Reeve J, Byng R. (2017). Realising the full potential of primary care: Uniting the 'two faces' of generalism. British Journal of General Practice, 67, pp. 292–293.

Reeve J, Cooper L. (2014). Rethinking how we understand individual healthcare needs for people living with long-term conditions: A qualitative study. Health and Social Care in the Community, 24, pp. 27–38.

Reeve J, et al. (2022). Deprescribing medicines in older people living with multimorbidity and polypharmacy: The TAILOR evidence synthesis. Health Technology Assessment, 26(32), pp. 1–148. https://www.journalslibrary.nihr.ac.uk/hta/AAFO2475#/abstract

Reeve E, Thompson W, Farrell B. (2017). Deprescribing: A narrative review of the evidence and practical recommendations for recognizing opportunities and taking action. European Journal of Internal Medicine 38, pp. 3–11.

Ridge K. (2021). National overprescribing review report. Department of Health and Social Care, UK Government.

Royal College of General Practitioners (RCGP). (2022). Fit for the Future: Retaining the GP Workforce. London: RCGP.

Tinetti ME, Fried T. (2004). The end of the disease era. American Journal of Medicine, 116, pp. 179–185.

Unal et al. (2004). Explaining the decline in coronary heart disease mortality in England and Wales between 1981 and 2000. Circulation, 109, p. 1101.7.

World Health Organisation (WHO). (1978). Declaration of Alma Ata. https://www.who.int/publications/i/item/WHO-EURO-1978-3938-43697-61471

CHAPTER 6

Medical generalism, now!

···

Healthcare needs medical generalism. Medical generalism is the expertise of whole person medicine. Lewis (2013) summarised the arguments for whole person medicine in an editorial calling for reform to Health Policy (see Box 6.1). Healthcare systems around the world continue to employ people with generalist skills – including general practitioners and doctors working in general internal medicine. Policy leaders, both in the UK and internationally, continue to call for a culture shift in healthcare to better recognise the person at the centre of care delivery. We need Medical Generalism, Now!

Where things break down is in knowing how we can deliver high-quality medical generalist care consistently and at scale in front-line, everyday healthcare settings. That is what I have been focusing on in this book – what changes do we need, and how do we put them into practice. My discussions have recognised three key areas for change: the need to implement an extended vision of whole person healthcare, address the missing element of knowledge work for practice and develop the infrastructure needed to support this model of care (Figure 6.1).

In Chapter 5, I described an *extended united vision for whole person healthcare* recognising that whole person healthcare systems need to deliver two distinct but complementary forms of clinical practice: generalist and specialist care. Some people, and some individual's healthcare problems, need condition-specific healthcare. Healthcare systems have a wealth of experience and expertise in delivering this 'specialist' – or what my international colleagues describe as 'partialist' healthcare. But for a growing proportion of people using Western

DOI: 10.1201/9781003297222-6

BOX 6.1 THE NEED FOR GENERALISM

[S]pecialization, which for all of its vast expansion of deep knowledge and therapeutic wizardry has not translated into universally improved care... There is strong evidence that the quality of care for many patients with multiple long-term conditions is substandard, resulting in diminished quality of life, avoidable complications and costly preventable hospital admissions. The risk of fragmentation and therapeutic complexity can cancel out the benefit derived from focusing on specific conditions... [T]he arguments in favour of a return to generalism have gathered steam.

(Lewis 2013)

---

healthcare, that care is not enough. People living with complex multimorbidity, the burden of chronic illness including the impact of healthcare, and those living with persistent physical symptoms that cannot be adequately explained or addressed by specialist healthcare all need a different approach. They need whole person medicine. So a

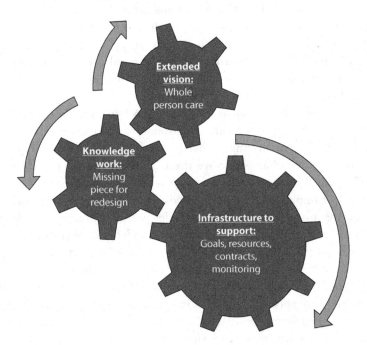

Figure 6.1   Three areas for change needed to embed advanced generalism in everyday practice.

person-centred healthcare system (WHO 2023) needs to be able to provide both specialist (condition specific) and generalist (whole person) assessment and management of illness problems.

In Chapter 2, I described how whole person medical clinical practice differs from condition-specific medical practice. Specifically, I outlined the *knowledge work of whole person, medical generalist practice.* This is the work needed to create, use and critique tailored, whole person understanding and management of illness in context. Generalist medicine is a distinct form of clinical reasoning – grounded in scientific practice, but different to the scientific reasoning and practice of evidence-based medicine (EBM).

I have described examples of generalist practice and reasoning in everyday work, but also recognised that front-line clinicians report multiple barriers to doing this knowledge work in practice. Take medical training as one example. Our current teaching recognises two forms of clinical reasoning: Intuitive (Type 1) and Analytical (Type 2 hypothetico-deductive) reasoning (see Chapter 2). Students of medicine are introduced to both, supported to develop the skills of Type 2 reasoning, so that with time and experience they may develop Type 1. Yet, students are not systemically introduced to the reasoning of generalist medicine – to inductive reasoning. I have proposed that we need to extend our current teaching models to include this third type of reasoning: Analytical (Inductive) reasoning. Yet, I also recognised that it isn't just students who need this support. My research has repeatedly described that a lack of understanding, skills and confidence in the knowledge work of whole person medicine is a problem not just for medical students but across all career stages and professional groups. In Chapter 5, I described how our CATALYST programme is remotivating GPs by helping them develop the knowledge work skills of advanced generalist practice.

Barriers to the knowledge work of generalist practice exist right across our healthcare systems. In Chapter 1, I recognised four factors: perceived lack of permission for generalist care, prioritisation of the work involved, skills and confidence in the tasks of generalist care and feedback to support and enable trusted best practice. Tackling these barriers means *addressing the infrastructure* barriers to practice. Training healthcare professionals differently is part of what is needed, but we also need to change the context (practice settings) in which they work and the policy that shapes and defines the work that they do.

In this penultimate chapter, I want to consider how we could practically start to introduce those changes and describe what that could look like on the ground. I'm going to explore that using the example of UK general practice. It's a context I know well and am therefore able to develop the applied discussions. But as I write, it is also a sector at crisis point. In 2016, Roland and Everington stated that 'if primary care fails, then the NHS fails'. We stand at a crossroads in healthcare redesign in the UK. To prevent the catastrophe that Professor Roland described, we need to focus – now – on primary care. So that's where I start in this chapter.

6.1 STARTING IN PRIMARY CARE

There are many reasons to choose primary care as the starting point for thinking about healthcare redesign. In the UK, 90% of healthcare happens in primary care – hence, Professor Roland's warning of the impact if it fails. Getting reform right in primary care will therefore have a major impact on the NHS as a whole. Secondly, my vision of whole person healthcare aligns with the definition of primary care: the provision of continuous, coordinated, comprehensive, accessible, *person-centred* healthcare (WHO 2023). Strong primary care has been shown to deliver efficient, effective and equitable healthcare (Kringos et al. 2013). So if we strengthen whole person (generalist) care, we strengthen primary care and therefore the delivery of equitable, effective and efficient healthcare. But perhaps my main reason for grounding this discussion in the primary care setting is that my team and I are already delivering change in this context, and with early signals of a positive impact. Chapters 3 through 5 described the impact of changing primary care knowledge work in the context of individual case studies. The next goal is to scale those up to deliver wider impact.

I have been discussing these ideas with colleagues across the primary care sector for some time. Their challenge to me was to describe the practical changes that could deliver the knowledge work of Medical Generalism, Now! They told me I needed to offer people a clear description and justification of what we were trying to do (what is this thing called knowledge work?), together with practical support for how it could be done.

To tackle the first, I set up WiseGP. WiseGP is a collaboration between the UK Royal College of General Practitioners and the Society for Academic Primary Care. WiseGP supports general practice, not just GPs. It exists to promote, advance and sustain the knowledge work of advanced professional practice for modern front-line general practice. Its goal is to help clinicians develop confidence in being able to use, but also move beyond, biomedical scientific evidence to safely and effectively tailor the healthcare they deliver to the needs of the individuals, families and communities they work with. The WiseGP community provides resources that can help practitioners recognise and value the advanced knowledge work of their everyday practice, and take part in activities to extend their skills and confidence. We have a growing network of people using WiseGP.

In this chapter, I want to build on those WiseGP beginnings, adding in the elements developed in this book, to propose a Wise Blueprint for a new model of general practice. My vision of Wise General Practice is grounded in the united vision of whole person healthcare described in Chapter 5, and incorporating the knowledge work of complex practice that has been the thread throughout this book. The blueprint intentionally offers a framework supporting implementation rather than an off-the-shelf tool to deliver. Implementation requires the knowledge work of professional practice – creating, critiquing and using knowledge in context – and needs to happen in context, and in partnership. Those conversations have started in the areas where I work. This chapter describes that framework so that you can consider if and how it works in your context. My account recognises the need for three layers of change – in Policy, Practice and People.

6.2 WISE POLICY

My blueprint for Wise General Practice starts with proposed changes to healthcare policy. Healthcare policy sets out the vision for healthcare systems, describing the plans for action, and the anticipated goals (impact) that will be achieved as a result. My Wise Blueprint proposes changes to both vision and impact.

Vision

UK healthcare policy is currently built on a vision of disease management, supported by guideline defined care. As healthcare needs in the population expand, escalate and so outstrip service capacity, focus has turned to seeking better integration of the multiple elements of condition-focused care to achieve more efficient delivery of care. Yet, there is no recognition in current policy of the need for, and potential benefit of, advanced generalist care. The UK policy of integrated healthcare fails to recognise the extended vision of integrated care described in the United Generalism model discussed in Chapter 5. If we are to benefit from Medical Generalism, Now! we need to update the vision in our healthcare policy.

We therefore need a new Wise Policy supporting an extended vision of whole person healthcare. I described the vision in Chapter 1 – to promote and enable health as a resource for living, and not an end in itself. This defines our understanding of 'best care' and becomes the framework used by healthcare professionals, patients and managers to make very practical decisions about the daily work they do.

Every professional wants to deliver the best care they can; every patient reasonably expects to get best care. If we define best care by the management of disease, it inevitably shapes the work that people do. Professionals prioritise, and patients receive, disease care. If the work of general practice is rewarded (financially and in other ways such as league tables) by, for example, how well it finds people with high blood pressure and puts them on guideline-defined care pathways, this is the work that people do. Let's imagine Sergio comes to see his GP to discuss a health concern that is interfering with his everyday life – making him feel anxious and stopping him getting on with things. In the waiting room, the practice invites people to check their blood pressure so it can be recorded in their notes. Sergio checks his and tells the receptionist. His blood pressure is found to be high and he is whisked off to see the practice nurse for it to be checked again. Sergio then goes in to see his GP, but all attention is now on his BP rather than the original reason he came. The attention of the healthcare system has been diverted to addressing the blood pressure issue rather than the problem he came with. At best, Sergio now has two problems to deal with, his blood pressure and the original issue. At worst, all the attention might be diverted to managing his blood pressure leaving Sergio still dealing with his original concern on his own.

There may be good reasons, at a whole population level, to be opportunistically looking to screen for hypertension (although also a number of epidemiological as well as person-centred reasons to be cautious too). But we are now starting to recognise that our continued efforts to seek out and manage disease risk factors are contributing to iatrogenic harm, including escalating health service use, and distracting attention from alternative approaches to managing health and health risk (e.g., see the discussion of Capewell's work in Chapter 5). We are so busy seeking out new disease that our resources are distracted from whole person care that focuses on health for daily living – building the individual and social capital of healthy people and health populations. So my Wise Policy supporting Medical Generalism, Now! describes a revised goal for healthcare that focuses on whole person health for daily living. By effectively defining best care as whole person care, this revised policy offers permission to front-line practitioners to tailor care to the needs of the individual in context.

My discussion of Normalisation Process Theory in Chapter 2 reminds us that healthcare professionals need more than permission to act, but also to be supported in recognising the impact of their actions. This feedback is a key element in enabling them to continue in their daily work, especially for work that is complex and challenging. So my Wise Policy needs to not only give permission for whole person care, but also to describe what impact we expect to see as a result of our actions and so how we can monitor the care we deliver. It needs to offer a meaningful framework that guides both health professionals and service users in their everyday healthcare work.

One of the reasons that condition-focused medicine has become so dominant in new public management run healthcare systems is that it is easy to define and measure best practice and success. A policy vision of, for example, reducing cardiovascular disease, can be readily monitored: seeing the impact of our policy and so be encouraged to continue in our actions, or indeed to change direction. The problem with a vision of promoting 'health for daily living' is that it is too vague to be useful. Critics may describe it as academic blue sky speak, but not useful for the day-to-day reality of running a healthcare system. Whole person healthcare can only become a reality if I can also describe a framework by which it can be put into practice and shown to make a difference. So how do we do that?

Impact

One approach would be to simply adapt our current models of practice to include a new, additional, outcome of whole person care. This would need us to first develop a suitable tool to measure health for daily living.

Many people have tried to develop tools that capture at least some elements of this concept. There are a host of 'person-centred' outcome tools now available. Most have been developed for research, and so are not designed practically to be used in the busy setting of clinical practice. In 20 years of looking, I have never found a tool that, for me, captures the complexity of outcomes from advanced generalist practice. It takes years to develop a new tool. Some people have told me it just isn't possible to measure generalist care. Back to the drawing board then …

Perhaps the answer to our dilemma comes instead from the core idea that threads through this book – the principles of knowledge work and broadening the scope of professional reasoning. The suggestion that we need a tool to measure the impact of healthcare on our expected outcomes is based on the deductive reasoning of specialist clinical practice and EBM. It assumes we can define a 'correct' goal and so statistically measure how close we are to achieving that. What if we turn instead to the inductive reasoning of advanced generalist practice? How could that help us with assessing the impact of our healthcare policy and vision?

Advanced generalist reasoning, grounded in inductive practice, does not rely on a single measure of outcome. The physician using advanced generalist practice works to explore and explain whole person illness. They create tailored understanding of an individual illness experience in context, use this explanation to implement a plan for action, and then follow up and evaluate what happens. This 'trial and learn' approach offers new information and, potentially, revised understanding of the problem. It is an iterative learning process. Gabbay and le May (2011) describe general practice teams creating practice-based evidence, or knowledge-in-practice-in-context, to support their daily clinical work (see Chapter 2). Can we do the same for the practice- and system-level aspects of our work?

The simple answer is no, not at the moment. Our healthcare systems are not designed to do so. We fund general practice to deliver items of service defined by external evidence and targets, and expect that practices collect and present data to show they have met those targets (see the discussion of PACT in Chapter 4). Yet, many voices have suggested that healthcare management needs to change (Learmonth and Harding 2004). The Wise Blueprint supports that change by explicitly bringing knowledge work activities into the way we monitor healthcare quality at a practice level. It requires a shift in understanding of general practice from a service delivery model to a learning organisation approach. Learning organisations are 'skilled at creating, acquiring and [using] knowledge, and at modifying [their] behaviour to reflect the new knowledge and insights [gained]' (Garvin 1993). Within the Wise Blueprint, we explicitly contract with local services to undertake the work to define, deliver and evaluate whole-person-care-in-context. This would allow us to end the micro-management of general practice criticised by the recent Health Select Committee (2022) government report and also adequately support and resource the alternative approach needed.

So how might front-line general practice explore, explain and evaluate whether it is delivering whole person care supporting health for daily living? If that question came to my research team, we'd start by asking ourselves what changes might we expect to see from this new approach, and how would we explore whether that has happened? We'd ask, what data could we collect to look for both the changes we are expecting, as well as others we haven't thought of yet. We would also consider questions about how we plan to analyse the data to create explanations and evaluation – I'll come back to that. But essentially, we'd be creating an initial explanatory impact model that we'd plan to try out (explore and explain) and learn from (evaluate) in practice.

Using that thought process, and drawing on the case studies and discussions I have presented in this book, I have described a draft Impact model for the Wise Blueprint (shown in Figure 6.2). To achieve our Wise Vision of an extended vision of whole person healthcare supporting health for daily living, we plan to work with primary care teams to embed the knowledge work of advanced generalist care into everyday practice. The changes we'd expect to see as a result would be improved health for daily living for individuals and communities (Chapter 1), reduced healthcare and illness burden (Chapter 3) and improved clinician motivation and morale (Chapter 5). All of which contribute to delivering strong primary care (continuous, comprehensive, coordinated, accessible person-centred care) and

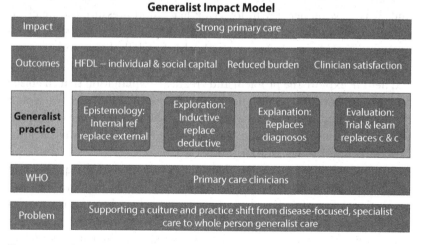

Generalist Impact Model

Impact	Strong primary care			
Outcomes	HFDL – individual & social capital	Reduced burden		Clinician satisfaction
Generalist practice	Epistemology: Internal ref replace external	Exploration: Inductive replace deductive	Explanation: Replaces diagnosos	Evaluation: Trial & learn replaces c & c
WHO	Primary care clinicians			
Problem	Supporting a culture and practice shift from disease-focused, specialist care to whole person generalist care			

Figure 6.2   The anticipated impact of the Wise Blueprint (derived from the generalist impact model).

so to improving the efficiency, effectiveness and equity of primary healthcare provision (Kringos et al. 2013). An extended primary care team could be supported to design ways to collect and analyse data to critically examine each element of that model. The analysis would describe what impact was being achieved, what was working well and what needs to be amended. Essentially, we have a model for a learning organisation.

Evaluating burden

To show you how a draft impact model can support a learning organisation approach, let's take a closer look at the three outcomes of advanced generalist practice that I have suggested here. I'll start with an outcome of a reduction in (iatrogenic) burden. In Chapter 1, I described how some of the everyday burden experienced by people living with long-term conditions comes from the effect of healthcare. This impacts not only on their daily lives, but also on their use of health services. Reducing burden is an important outcome for healthcare.

Optimising medical management can reduce disease burden, but that can come at the cost of increased treatment burden. Balancing optimisation of care and avoidance of treatment burden may require compromise. We can see a simple example of this when we consider the use of medicines to prevent future cardiovascular risk. Let's consider Sally, an 80-year-old woman living with heart failure. She takes a beta-blocker (bisoprolol) to optimise her long-term survival. As she gets older, she finds it is slowing her down, lowering her blood pressure too much so she has dizzy spells. In conversation with her GP, she decides the negative impact of the medicine on her health for daily living today is not justified by the potential longer-term benefit to her length of life. Sally and her GP explore the problem and create an explanation that the bisoprolol is not benefiting Sally enough to continue it. They agree on a plan to stop it, but also put in place a plan to evaluate the change – with the potential to revise the decision. Tailored care has reduced Sally's healthcare burden, for today at least.

So how would we recognise that in an evaluation of the quality and effectiveness of healthcare? There are research tools that can measure perceptions of burden, but alone they are unlikely to be sensitive enough to pick up significant change. Our experience from running the Complex Needs work (Chapter 4) was that changes that are clinically significant for patients and clinicians are not necessarily matched by statistically significant changes in the numbers used to measure care. So we might need to use a range of different data sources to explore the effect of care, use our knowledge work skills to create explanation (practice-based evidence) in context, and so review and revise (evaluate) our plans for both care delivery and ongoing learning. We can quickly see that this has become a significant task to do. We need to consider what data sources are useful, collect and analyse the data and then interpret our findings.

One response might be to suggest this is 'taking clinicians away from front-line patient care' and that cost is too great to pay. We have (external) systems in place that monitor routine care; systems that are 'good enough' for a lot of what we do. We can exception report someone like Sally from those assessments. We shouldn't use clinical time and expertise for 'monitoring' healthcare. Certainly, I would accept that our existing systems may be 'good enough' for monitoring Routine Specialist care (as identified in the United Generalism model in Chapter 5) – and therefore a good proportion of the work that we do. But, as I have described throughout this book, this approach is not enough to support advanced generalist practice and therefore a growing body of our daily work. For patients in the Advanced Generalist quadrant of our United Generalism model, we need a different approach to evaluating the delivery of care. We need to extend the knowledge work used in individual patient care to support evaluation of practice population-level care too. Crucially, we must recognise this as an integral part of front-line patient care – the work to create the knowledge-in-practice-in-context (Gabbay and le May 2011) that enables us to deliver extended whole person care on the ground. We need to both design knowledge work into the working week of everyday practice, and resource it properly. In this way, we create the learning organisation model I have described and embed knowledge work actions into the routine, prioritised everyday work of general practice.

Evaluating individual and social capital

The second outcome on the Wise Blueprint impact model refers to the expectations of healthcare. Advanced generalist care supports a culture shift in healthcare – from 'fixing' to 'managing' a problem. Healthcare rarely fixes. As Voltaire is credited with saying, 'the art of medicine consists of amusing the patient while nature cures the disease'. In my own research, patient participants have told me that they believe their medicines are 'keeping them alive' – including patients on cardiovascular primary prevention medicines (Reeve and Cooper 2014). Embedding advanced generalist healthcare into everyday practice would mean explicitly working with patients to recognise optimised health for daily living as an expected and legitimate outcome of care. Could we then expect to see an impact on how people use health services (and indeed wider societal resources) to improve their health? I introduced the concept of candidacy (perceived eligibility for healthcare) in Chapter 3 as part of a wider discussion about access. We might predict that introducing advanced generalist practice could impact people's understanding and use of health services within all three areas of candidacy, concordance and recursivity.

With over 30 million GP consultations per month currently happening in UK general practice, it might take a while to see an impact on these population-level numbers. But one (routine) data source we could look at could be the number of consultations that an individual patient has had in the last, say, 3–6 months. Five years ago in the UK, the average number of consultations with your GP was about four a year. Today, I am seeing many patients who have had four consultations with the practice in the last month. Some of that reflects the fragmentation of healthcare services meaning people need to make multiple contacts to get through to the care they need. Plans for integrated healthcare systems may help with that. But some of that growth is caused by a failure to offer united whole person healthcare. We treat ever more 'conditions' but fail to deliver the whole person explanation and management of illness in context that people need.

We have the data systems to monitor at practice level who many consultations patients are having. I would propose that if we were to implement the new Wise Blueprint policy, we could expect to see a change (drop) in consultation patterns and a de-escalation of healthcare use. We already have the data sources we could use to explore those changes. We would need to embed the resources to support the work to explain and evaluate the data.

Clinician satisfaction

My third suggestion for expected change might raise some eyebrows because it focuses not on patients, but on healthcare staff. I propose that a vision of best practice for care must recognise the needs of staff as well as service users, because without staff, we can't have a good healthcare system. We have a workforce crisis in UK healthcare. Staff are burning out because of the sheer volume of work. But as I discussed in Chapter 5, our experiences from the CATALYST programme demonstrate that we also need to reset our vision of what we're trying to do. GPs joining us on the CATALYST programme describe being overwhelmed by the task of rescuing people from the disease river. Yet, our evaluation shows that by helping GPs develop a vision of their role as advanced generalist knowledge workers, they describe a new sense of meaning, mastery and motivation in their everyday work. So if we were to scale this approach and introduce knowledge work principles into general routine, the third 'outcome' I would expect to see from introduction of the Wise Blueprint is a change in workforce motivation.

In summary: A wise policy

The Wise Policy therefore recognises two elements: an extended vision of whole person healthcare (United Generalism) supporting health for daily living, enabled through the knowledge work of advanced generalist practice within a learning organisation. I have proposed three outcomes that we might expect to observe if we were to introduce this policy: reduced burden on patients, change in expectations of and use of healthcare, and workforce satisfaction. I have explored how we might start to evaluate those changes; and so create new learning organisation model for practice able to use knowledge created in context to modify its behaviour (Garvin 1993). I have acknowledged potential concerns about whether this work is a 'legitimate' part of front-line clinical practice. Therefore, I will next look more closely at the implications for how we design and deliver Wise Practices.

6.3 WISE PRACTICE

As I write, UK general practice is at breaking point. Staff, patients and the service are overwhelmed. The priority for most people at the moment is to make care manageable and safe, for both patients and staff. Certainly, there are conversations about how we can recruit more staff. But the immediate pressures mean most people are asking what can we (safely) stop doing? Any suggestion about introducing something new will be met with the question: What does this replace? In that context, where does knowledge work fit? How does it help – indeed, can it help?

I start by recognising that there are two parts to thinking about general practice change. Firstly, what do we want future care to look like; and secondly, how can we get there from the point we find ourselves in now. The work it will take to transition from where we are now to where we want to be is significant. It would take a whole separate book

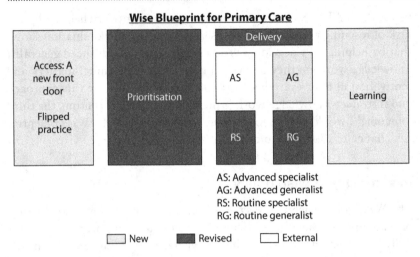

Figure 6.3   Describing the new Wise Practice.

to describe the process of change and how we get there. I want to start here by thinking about the potential endpoint – where we are trying to get to. I will be drawing on the ideas I have developed in this book, to develop and describe a prototype for a new model of extended whole person general practice care. My aim is to spark a conversation, but also to plan a pilot study. I want to start some knowledge-work-in-context to create, use and critique this new model of general practice. All of which lays the foundations for the work to transition from where we are now, to where we could be.

My prototype for a new Wise Practice is summarised in Figure 6.3. Each block recognises a distinct body of work to do. Each will need to be described in detail and in context, so that it can be adequately resourced and planned into a practical 'working week' for front-line care. The concepts presented in this book provide the building blocks for implementing this model, and for evaluating the impact on Wise Policy goals of shifting culture, reducing burden and revitalising a workforce. There are four elements in this model: Flipped Practice, Whole Person Prioritisation, United Care and Learning.

Access: A new front door

In Chapter 3, I introduced our work on the Flipped Consultation – an approach supporting, amongst other things, the use of the advanced Generalist Gatekeeper or Guru role. This approach has the potential to deliver against our Wise Policy goal to reduce the burden of over-medicalisation. The Flipped Consultation came out of our work on the BOUNCEBACK project – a model in which we welcomed non-medical health expertise into the general practice setting. BOUNCEBACK was the beginning of developing a Flipped Practice model. My proposal now is to develop and extend that work further.

Since the introduction of general practice in the NHS, the GP has been the first point of call for patients seeking primary medical care. For a proportion of patients, that remains necessary and important; but it is not the only approach. Here, I want to explore how we can safely and systematically introduce change into our redesign of general practice.

As Iona Heath highlighted in her Harveian lecture (Chapter 3), the public are continuously managing significant volume of illness work that they never bring to healthcare services. I start by not only acknowledging that, but actively seeking to celebrate and support that work further through the way we design our healthcare systems. As I discussed in Chapter 1, individuals and communities are actively engaged in work that draws on their individual creative capacity to maintain daily living, including in the face of illness related disruption. Communities offer a host of additional support in this work through the work of friends and families as well as charities, voluntary groups and wider. Some of these community activities are becoming newly recognised and formalised through the introduction of so-called Social Prescribing in the NHS. The aim is to make social networks of support more visible and accessible to people with health-related needs that they might otherwise present to their GP, but then not get the help they are looking for. By broadening the offer of the community resource that is general practice, to better match the range of needs presented by community members, we may contribute to de-escalation of healthcare use and reduced burden of healthcare.

So my first proposal is to develop a new *front door* to practice; a front door that recognises, by adequately resourcing, the expertise of the community. It is a front door which grounds a practice in its community setting. Developing the door requires practices to work with communities to agree the goals and priorities for local healthcare – what it can, and can't, do to support health for living. (We'll touch on this again in Chapter 7 when Dr Hjorleifsson talks about the work they are doing on this in Norway.)

This new front door will extend the Flipped Consultation model from Chapter 3 into a Flipped Practice model. The practice will work with communities to find new ways to respond to problems that are disrupting daily living, perceived to be health related, and may benefit from a non-medical response – working on the illness rather than the disease side of the gate described by Iona Heath (Chapter 3). Our key goal would be to optimise the visibility and access to an appropriate range of resources to support health for daily living; optimised by the opportunity to use and learn from these approaches. In this way, we hope to effectively address the warning from Illich (1973) – the unintended harm created by over medicalising every aspect of our daily lives.

This will not be an easy goal to deliver. It needs both practitioners and patients to potentially change the way they deal with health issues. In the UK, we have seen attempts by individual practices to start these conversations with their registered patients in recent months. Practices have published letters to their communities, including in social media, asking people to use the service differently. Often these initiatives have created bad press and antagonism with local communities. They have been perceived as blaming patients for the problems that practices face, suggesting that the problem is only down to patient behaviour. That is certainly not the message behind the Flipped Practice idea, and indeed the models of care we used in BOUNCEBACK and wider. But we will clearly need to think carefully about how we'd implement a Flipped Practice.

The use of an assets-based, rather than deficit-based, community engagement is one approach that would resonate with the cultural shift described here. Past community engagement approaches have been deficit focused – undertaking 'needs assessment' to meet externally defined 'gaps'. For example, services might define smoking rates as the local priority. Measurement of teenage smoking rates highlights higher rates in one area and so describes a 'need' to strengthen smoking cessation services in this community. This is a deficit-based assessment built on an external definition of best care. By contrast, an asset-based approach might instead work with a community and so recognise a strong youth development programme in an area. The agreed priority is to work with the community to understand how it can be developed and sustained. The community and the service both invest in work to develop this resource and understand the impact on community health. We are using (inductive) knowledge work principles to support community health development to the benefit of individuals, communities and the health service. By engaging local communities in the knowledge work to explore and explain the impact of the new service, we develop shared understanding of the value and use of the service. Another example of using knowledge work to achieve whole person healthcare.

Prioritisation

Our flipped approach may help some of our patients to find and utilise non-medical support to help restore and optimise their health for daily living. Others will need general practice care. The next stage in our Wise Practice model is to describe how we get the right person to the right sort of care.

Care allocation – aiming to get the right patient to the right member of the extended clinical team – is nothing new in general practice. It is, however, a hot topic as the service looks to deal with both the after effects of the COVID-19 lockdown, and escalating demand. We have seen introduction of a host of digital tools to try and improve the demand management and allocation processes. To date, efforts have focused on two elements: assessing risk and speeding up diagnosis. Systems have embedded tools to ensure patients at acute risk of harm are flagged to appropriate urgent services. Here, I want to focus on the diagnosis element.

Digital triage of patients is pretty routine in most general practices now. Patients are asked a series of questions aimed at better understanding their problem and so assessing the urgency of their request and who they need to help them (e.g., a clinician or administrator). Many of the new digital tools also seek to collect data that may help frame a clinical diagnosis. From a service perspective, the ideal would be to design a system where patients can input their symptoms, algorithms accurately diagnose the problem, and the patient is directed to the optimal management approach – whether a prescription or a referral. The goal is to improve the speed, efficiency and accuracy of medical diagnosis and management.

Of course, this assumes that the patient's problem can be dealt with using biomedical, hypothetico-deductive reasoning. In Medical Generalism, Now! I have focused on the growing proportion of our patient population for whom this disease approach is insufficient or won't work. Extended whole person healthcare described within United Generalism describes a need to use both generalist and specialist care to provide whole person care to an individual. The digital tools we have so far may help us with managing specialist care, but they are not designed to support inductive generalist care. We still need to find ways to help us identify the patients who need more than a single condition-focused approach.

Until recently, this complex work of picking up the person who 'didn't fit' and matching them to the right clinician was most commonly done by trained reception staff. Experienced staff have become highly skilled in recognising and directing patients (How often has one of your reception-ists rung you to say 'Mrs Manjula popped in to say she's just got a water infection, but there's something not right – she doesn't normally come in. Can you see her?'). We will continue to rely on that expertise for some time to come, I suspect. As I described in Chapter 3, Etz and colleagues also highlighted the importance of the under-recognised prioritisation role of the generalist in sorting, ranking and negotiating the importance of multiple elements of healthcare need presented by individuals. This includes the ability to identify when patients need a disease-focused (specialist) approach, or a whole person (generalist) approach. There are multiple ways in which current general practice makes decisions about how it allocates care to patients, and we want to hold on to the best of these.

I am also exploring with colleagues if there are ways that we can also adapt digital technology to help us with that allocation process. Asking, can we identify data that flags someone as needing general-ist, rather than condition-specific, input. The obvious flags would be reported burden, as just discussed, or predicted burden identified perhaps by looking at the number of long-term conditions someone lives with, or medicines they take every day. UK general practice now routinely records frailty status. But our analysis from the Complex Needs project (Chapter 5) suggested that 'routine' general practice data related to diagnoses and medication may not be enough to recognise people in need of advanced generalist care. In that work, we were able to identify some factors which seemed to identify people who ben-efited from the advanced generalist approach compared with routine care. But these were usually non-medical factors, things not routinely recorded in patients' clinical records. For example, we noted that lev-els of social support, changes in circumstances and often sub-clinical levels of distress and mental health were key predictors. I have started a conversation with digital providers to consider how we might build those elements into digital triage tools. I have also previously suggested another marker of vulnerability to burden and health-related disrup-tion to daily living, namely frequency of health service use. Frequent use of and contact with services suggests that needs are not being met and so flags a potential need to see an advanced generalist practitioner.

Local teams will be able to identify additional markers relevant to their own communities.

Once again, this discussion highlights the need for new resource in practice to support the knowledge work needed to create, use and critique and amend this knowledge-in-practice-in-context. Introducing Generalist Prioritisation is dependent on the introduction of the Learning Organisation component in Wise Policy.

Delivery

My third suggestion is to redesign service delivery around the four types of care described within the United Generalism model that I outlined in Chapter 5. The United Generalism model recognises distinct models of care in each of its four quadrants – three of which are offered in the general practice setting. Specialist and generalist quadrants use different skill sets and resources to assess and deliver care need. Reviews of best practice in settings outside of healthcare (both business and education) have repeatedly described that 'unbundling and re-bundling' the daily activities of an organisation can improve efficiency, effectiveness and – perhaps paradoxically – creativity and flexibility (Hagel and Singer 1999; Czierniewicz 2018). Yet, the typical GP working day still reflects a view of the GP as a 'jack of all trades'. In a morning surgery, the clinician can be expected to move swiftly and repeatedly between specialist and generalist, as well as routine and advanced decision-making approaches. If this was possible to do effectively in years gone past, it certainly no longer feels possible to do safely, and satisfactorily, given both the volume and complexity of work.

So the third element of the Wise Practice model seeks to unbundle and rebundle the everyday work of practice into the four United Generalism quadrants. Patients are prioritised (matched) to the best starting quadrant. Clinicians are allocated to work spaces according to their skill sets and expertise. Of course, there would need to be scope for people to move between quadrants, guided by the exploration and understanding of their problem that took place. We would expect that allocation processes wouldn't always be perfect, and we know that the problem someone presents with often masks an underlying issue. We'd also be expecting to evaluate the impact of these changes: on reducing burden for patients, and improving clinician satisfaction.

Once again, there is some significant work to be done to define and develop these new bundles of activity, and to match them to the prioritisation elements previously discussed. We'd need to look carefully at the training of, and resources for, clinicians working in each of these new spaces. The Learning Organisation element of the Wise Blueprint remains key.

Learning

The fourth component of the Wise Blueprint is a dedicated practice-level work stream focused on Learning. As I have been discussing throughout this book, whole person medicine grounded in inductive reasoning generates explanations that are reasonable, best interpretations of the data – that are probable but not certain. Evaluation of the explanation – its impact and usefulness – is a fundamental part of defining and delivering quality (best) practice. A Wise Practice therefore needs to have learning processes actively embedded in their daily work – not a bolt on as in the PACT evaluation (Chapter 4) but an integral part of the delivery of care. All parties need to be involved in this learning; although their specific roles in that process may differ.

Patients living with long-term conditions are learning every day. They are the experts in their own personal experience of whatever condition(s) they have. In Chapter 1, I described some of the research that has been done to describe the creative capacity of individuals as they learn to adapt and live with their new condition. Perhaps the most important thing that we can design into healthcare here is to recognise its role as support and facilitator of that learning – ideally helping learning, but certainly not disrupting it. As people live with the disruptive impact of illness, they learn to manage that impact. That learning shapes all aspects of how they subsequently access healthcare. This includes when and whether they see themselves as needing to contact a health practitioner (candidacy), how they work with health practitioners to manage the problem (concordance) and how they engage with and use healthcare in the future (recursivity). The Wise Practice recognises one part of its role is to help patients develop their understanding of how and when to use healthcare in the future. This element of the Learning role of Wise Practice feeds in turn into the Access element – helping to shape how the patient uses the service in future. This is work that already happens in everyday general practice, but it is hidden work – not designed into the working day for clinicians and the resources available for patient care. The Wise Practice model seeks to make this work explicit and, therefore, sustainable.

The Learning Organisational approach of the Wise Practice model explicitly recognises knowledge work activities as an integral part of the everyday work of a practice team. Knowledge work has always happened in general practice – but it is often hidden, under the radar and therefore not valued. Learning work has too long been seen as an 'added extra', nice to do even, but the first thing to get squeezed out when things get busy. Colleagues have often told me that ours is a 'practical discipline'. We get on with things – the rest is seen as 'too academic' and not part of the 'real job'. Building knowledge work into the everyday activities of general practice – making it part of the 'real job' – is key to achieving the Wise Policy vision of optimising health for daily living through the advanced knowledge work of whole person practice. It is a significant culture shift from current models of practice but it is also the shift called for in the Fuller's recent review of the future of UK general practice. As described in my discussion of the CATALYST project in Chapter 5, evidence suggests it is also an approach that may help us to tackle our workforce crisis.

To achieve Medical Generalism, Now! we need to explicitly design knowledge work into the routine daily activity of the general practice setting including the team of people who work there. That means supporting team members to develop and use knowledge work skills. In the next section, I focus on how we support development of Wise People.

6.4 WISE PEOPLE

At the heart of this new vision is strengthened capacity for the knowledge work of whole person care. Knowledge work happens in conversations (or consultations) with patients, in the way individuals and teams work to build and run practices and in the way societies use health systems to support their goals.

We have established processes and systems for the knowledge work of condition-focused specialist medicine – applied EBM operating within New Public Management systems (or as critics describe it, scientific bureaucratic medicine). This work has made an important contribution to improving healthcare delivery. However, in Medical Generalism, Now! I have argued that current knowledge work is not sufficient for modern health service needs. Specifically, I have recognised that the scope of knowledge work in healthcare is 'incomplete'. It fails to support the whole person focus of advanced generalist medicine, now internationally recognised as being necessary to address emerging health system challenges such as multimorbidity, treatment burden and persistent physical symptoms. In describing the clinical knowledge work of advanced generalist care, I recognised it as a mechanism to support decision making for complex problems. The knowledge work skills of advanced generalist practice also support the work needed to design, deliver and evaluate healthcare at the practice level. I have therefore suggested that these knowledge work skills are the missing piece in current efforts to reform and modernise healthcare.

We therefore need to enable people working within modern healthcare to develop, use and learn from the skills of advanced generalist knowledge work. We need a plan to develop and support Wise People. I have been working on just that challenge for a number of years – including in developing, running and evaluating the CATALYST programme, and establishing WiseGP. That work has demonstrated the need for (at least) two elements: training in knowledge work skills, but also ongoing support for knowledge work in action. I will consider both of those in the final section of this chapter.

Knowledge work skills: Developing the 4Es

We do not consistently and routinely train clinicians in the knowledge work skills of inductive practice. This leaves a significant gap in the tools available to front-line practitioners to manage both whole person clinical care, but also the challenges of complex practice development. The result is a healthcare system unable to deliver whole person healthcare. That needs to change.

When I was planning this book, I thought I would be writing a generalist version of David Sackett's book on EBM. I imagined a series of 'how to do' chapters that would walk the clinician step by step through the job of creating knowledge-in-context. Only once I began writing did I realise I was falling into the same trap we face in clinical practice. I was trying to simply replace one set of prescribed knowledge (a guideline on disease management) with another set (a guideline on person management).

My experience from the CATALYST programme showed me how and why I needed to think differently. As I discussed in Chapter 5, our research shows that CATALYST works not by telling people what to do. Instead we teach them how to work out what they can do – safely and effectively, including sharing that exploration and explanation with their patients. We help them explore, understand and so embrace the inherent variability (what some describe as uncertainty) that comes with that process. Yet, we also help them develop new frameworks for best practice that enable them to feel 'safe' working in this complex space – recognising the capacity to review and revise our understanding of a problem as part of the wisdom of practice. Rather than always assuming there is a right answer, we seek to develop a best answer and then develop it through a 'trial and learn' approach.

Perhaps one of the strongest lessons that CATALYST has taught me is the importance and value of engaging collective community in this work. To an extent, I am surprised that I am surprised. As a researcher, I would never consider embarking on a process of generating and using (scientific) knowledge on my own. Why am I surprised that as a clinician, the same rules apply? Knowledge work is a community activity – especially inductive knowledge work. This book seeks to stimulate curiosity, to offer a guide to support some creative learning. But this book cannot replace the community of practice work that is ultimately needed to develop understanding, skills, confidence and use of generalist knowledge work in action. That is perhaps the fundamental difference between this book and Sackett's.

However, as CATALYST demonstrates, knowledge work, and the skills of advanced generalist practice, can certainly be 'taught' – introduced, developed and applied through professional development activities. I would argue that any health professional who is taught the deductive approaches of EBM should also learn the inductive methods of generalist medicine. Modern medical practice relies not on what you know, but how you use what you know. Therefore, those practising medicine need to understand the principles and practice of the scientific methods that generate that knowledge. They need to understand the principles of how we can trust what we know (epistemology) and so be able create (or at least find), use and critique that knowledge *in context*.

CATALYST is showing us that this learning needs three elements: a clear account of the principles of practice; a real-world set of problems in which to critically and creatively use those principles; and a critical, creative supportive space in which to undertake that 'trial and learn' approach. I have been working on ways to make all three more widely available.

WiseGP is an initiative that seeks to introduce working professionals to the principles of knowledge work practice. Working with colleagues including Annabelle Machin, Emily Lyness, Johanna Reilly and James Bennett, we have developed a set of resources that introduce the principles and so help professionals start to develop their practical understanding of, and trust in, knowledge work in context. We have a free-to-access online learning programme (WISDOM) based on the principles of CATALYST. We are now looking to use what we've learned so far to work with colleagues to develop a consensus statement on

---

BOX 6.2 PROPOSED WISE LEARNING OBJECTIVES

1. To understand the overlap and distinction between whole person medicine and integrated specialist medicine.
2. To understand the Epistemological principles and practice of inductive practice and Interpretive Medicine – generating knowledge-in-context for clinical and extended professional practice.
3. To apply the epistemological principles of inductive and abductive reasoning to critically review and revise the knowledge-in-context generated (Exploration, Explanation and Evaluation).
4. To critically describe, discuss and evaluate the implications for patient, population and professional outcomes.

---

the learning objectives for a Wise Learning programme (see Box 6.2), along with potential resources to support each stage. We'd aim for this to help professional groups develop tailored learning programmes for their own disciplines. We'd anticipate that all healthcare professionals complete objectives 1 and 2 in their professional training. Those looking to deliver advanced generalist clinical care would be expected to cover all four.

For these objectives to be useful in driving in professional practice, patient care relies on them being translated into action and learning in context. For that, I propose the need for a Wise Hub.

Supporting knowledge work communities: A wise hub

The impact of CATALYST depends on having created a Wise Hub – a critical creative space in which to translate learning objectives and ideals into change on the ground. This depends on having three elements: Protected Space, Facilitated Knowledge Work tackling real-world problems and Collective exploration of the impact. Firstly, CATALYST creates a protected space for professionals to work in, outside of the day-to-day patient-contact work of daily practice. Secondly, CATALYST introduces an idea to support change – that of the knowledge work of professional practice. And thirdly, it applies the idea to a series of Problems faced by the CATALYST participants to help them critically explore, explain and evaluate ideas from their own daily practice – to undertake knowledge work in context.

CATALYST is changing both patient care and the experience of health professionals. We need to embed this way of working into the everyday design of modern primary care and everyday practice. But CATALYST also highlights the importance and benefit of collaborative action. Gabbay and le May's work (2011, 2023) on the development of mindlines (knowledge-in-context) focuses on the knowledge work activities taking part in a clinical practice. My work in CATALYST, and indeed WiseGP, recognises a profession wide activity done within communities of practice that extend beyond individual practices. CATALYST acts as a hub supporting knowledge work activity across a wider community. I propose that we need to build this approach into the Wise Blueprint model for future general practice with the creation of Wise Hubs. Each Wise Practice is engaged in its own knowledge work, but all are connected through and with a Wise Hub. The Hub acts as a stimulus and resource for the local knowledge work needed to develop, deliver and evaluate an extended vision of whole person primary care. Hubs support sharing of the wisdom and knowledge work of advanced generalist care.

6.5   MEDICAL GENERALISM, NOW!

This chapter potentially outlines a huge task ahead of us. It may feel too daunting – too hard. Maybe we should just carry on pulling people out of the river as best we can? Its hard work, but at least its familiar. Do we just hope for the best …?

Yet, there is a growing body of data, of research, of policy statements, and most of all of stories from patients and healthcare professionals that tells us more of the same is not an option.

So instead, I want to finish by returning to where I started – with the person, the individual needing healthcare. Whether they are juggling multiple long-term conditions, persistent physical symptoms that evade biomedical diagnoses or the burden of illness or healthcare, they need a health service that can work with them to help manage the impact of these health-related issues on the creative capacity and the work of daily living.

These people need clinicians who can help them understand and deal with their health- and illness-related burden. They need clinicians skilled, confident and supported in the knowledge work of advanced generalist practice. Their clinicians need the capacity to work beyond disease or guideline boundaries to manage undifferentiated and complex

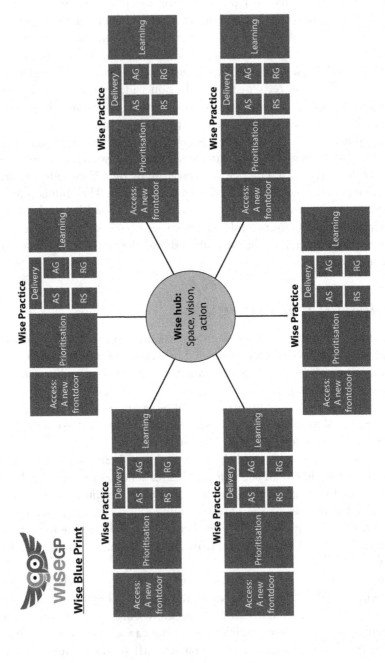

Figure 6.4   The Wise Blueprint – linking Wise Practices and Wise Hub.

care and so deliver tailored whole person exploration, explanation and evaluation of illness. These clinicians need to work in, and be supported by, a modern healthcare system that understands, values and supports this most complex form of care. To meet the needs of both patients and clinicians, healthcare systems need to change.

In this chapter, I described how we might address the system and practice barriers to advanced generalist practice and enable the professional knowledge work of modern advanced generalist care. I have discussed that there is more work to do to recognise and support the knowledge work of patients and the public – within the Flipped Practice and Learning elements of my Wise Blueprint.

As I near the end of this book, I am reflecting that it finishes in a different place to the one I imagined when I started writing it 2 years ago. The processes of exploring, explaining and evaluating the work of whole person healthcare, generalist care and modern medical practice – the knowledge work of writing a book – have challenged and developed my own thinking and practice. It has helped me to see the change that is both possible, and happening now. I hope that in reading this book, you too have been able to experience some of that.

A number of years ago, I was invited to give the Carl Moore lecture at McMaster University – the home of EBM. We agreed on a title of 'Time to Retire Evidence-Based Medicine'. When I started writing *Medical Generalism, Now*, I wondered if that lecture would be my focus for this story. Instead, it feels like I have been completing the story I started in that lecture. Writing and thinking about generalism has, in my experience, strengthened my understanding and appreciation of specialist medicine. Whole person healthcare needs both (United Generalism), but we also need to get better – individually, collectively and at systems level – at recognising when an individual needs which type of care.

Writing this book has also highlighted some essential 'missing pieces' in current efforts to redesign primary care, and indeed health services. As our health system struggles to cope with the demands placed on it, I am struck by the amount of work we are doing to try and deliver more of the same. We seem to have an almost blind faith in our ability to solve our problems by being more efficient. Indeed, we spend so much effort on improving efficiency that we forget to take that step back – an upstream look – to remember what it is we are ultimately trying to do, and so consider if and how we might do it differently.

So I would propose that we need to redesign health services around the knowledge work of healthcare practice – recognising the distinct process and value of both EBM and whole person Advanced Generalist Medicine. We need to re-organise our resources around those dual processes – with stratification (prioritisation) of patient needs, and clearer identification of professional skills for the different types of clinical work needed in each. We need to pay different and better attention to the four core practice-based elements needed to support knowledge work in practice: data, prioritisation, knowledge work and learning. All so that we can deliver a health system that enables the individual and societal benefit (capital) of enhancing health as a resource for living; rather than seeking to command and control disease.

An updated knowledge work framework for healthcare services delivers the culture shift called for in recent UK policy reports (e.g., Ridge 2021; Fuller 2022) as well as international calls from the World Health Organization. It has the potential to deliver the person-centred care called for in those policy initiatives, addressing the burden on patients. A knowledge work framework for health services addresses some of the burnout and burden experienced by professionals and so tackles one of our most urgent challenges – protecting our workforce. It offers parity of esteem in expertise – supporting recruitment but perhaps even more importantly retention of the existing expertise in our general practice workforce. A knowledge work framework offers new opportunities to support a culture shift in the academic sector too – valuing not just knowledge output, but also support for knowledge creation, use and critique. There will be challenges, for GPs, patients and health systems – in the same way the EBM caused upset. EBM has taken 30 years to embed into healthcare. I hope we can embed generalism quicker and achieve Medical Generalism, Now! But I accept it is a future goal too.

I came across the concept of knowledge work many years ago when exploring systems outside of healthcare. Indeed, I have often found ideas for dealing with the wicked problems I meet in everyday practice by going outside of healthcare. So I draw my discussion of medical generalism to a close by looking at the writing of Fred Kent whose work I came across some years ago. Kent is a city designer – designing spaces for humans, but in a very different context. In calling for people to rethink the design of urban spaces, he proposed that if we design cities for cars and traffic, we will simply generate more cars and traffic. But if we design cities for people, we get – well, spaces full of people.

Imagine what we could achieve if we applied the same thinking to designing healthcare.

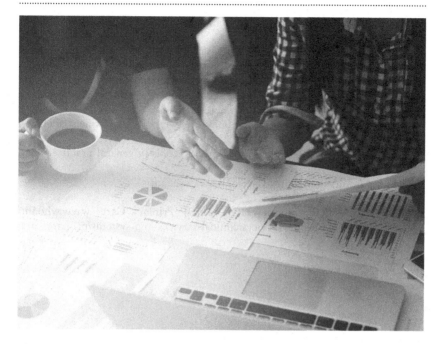

Planning spaces for people. The figure graphically illustrates the writing of Fred Kent, a city designer, who designs spaces for people to live in. He described that you can design cities for traffic flow and cars – and you will see lots of cars and traffic. Or you can design cities for people to be in – to walk in, to live in. Then, you will see people, living.

REFERENCES

Czierniewicz L. (2018). Unbundling and rebundling higher education in an era of inequality. EDUCAUSE Review. https://er.educause.edu/articles/2018/10/unbundling-and-rebundling-higher-education-in-an-age-of-inequality

Fuller C. (2022). Next Steps for Integrating Primary Care: Fuller Stocktake Report. NHS England.

Gabbay J, le May A. (2011). Practice-Based Evidence for Healthcare: Clinical Mindlines. London: Routledge.

Garvin DA. (1993). Building a learning organisation. Harvard Business Review. https://hbr.org/1993/07/building-a-learning-organization

Hagel J, Singer M. (1999). Unbundling the corporation. Harvard Business Review. https://hbr.org/1999/03/unbundling-the-corporation

Health Select Committee. (2022). The Future of General Practice. UK Parliament.

Illich I. (1973). Limits to Medicine: Medical Nemesis – The Expropriation of Health. Penguin Books.

Kringos D et al. (2013). The strength of primary care in Europe: An international comparative study. British Journal of General Practice, 63, pp. e742–750.

Lewis S. (2013). The two faces of generalism. Journal of Health Services Policy and Research, 19, pp. 1–2.

Learmonth M, Harding N. (2004). Unmasking Health Management: A Critical Text. New York: Nova Science Publishers.

Reeve J, Cooper L. (2014). Rethinking how we understand individual healthcare needs for people living with long-term conditions: A qualitative study. Health and Social Care in the Community, 24, pp. 27–38.

Ridge K. (2021). National overprescribing review report. Department of Health and Social Care, UK Government.

Roland M, Everington S. (2016). Tackling the crisis in general practice. BMJ, 352, p. i1942.

Society for Academic Primary Care: www.sapc.ac.uk

WISE GP: www.wisegp.co.uk

World Health Organisation (WHO). (2023). Primary Care. www.who.int/teams/integrated-health-services/clinical-services-and-systems/primary-care

CHAPTER 7

Medical generalism, everywhere?

....

7.1 INTRODUCING THE CONVERSATION

In this book, I have described a new vision for the delivery of medical generalist care at scale, and discussed the application in, and implications for, UK general practice. My ambition is that this work could support a global change in primary medical care. So I was interested to hear what my international colleagues think about the ideas. This chapter presents a first conversation with them.

It would need a whole new book to present a detailed discussion on the implementation of advanced generalist principles and practice in other national health systems – perhaps even a series of books. Yet, the ideas and concepts I have used in this book draw on professional writing and research from around the globe. An international community have been grappling with these issues for many decades. So the intention of this final chapter is to get a brief glimpse of where these generalist conversations are at for fellow primary care clinicians around the globe.

The initial plan was to have one big conversation. My goal was to invite people who have been writing and speaking on generalist practice to join a round table, virtual discussion. The challenges created by both international clocks and busy diaries meant that, in reality, this was done as three conversations. I edited those into one narrative – a 'virtual' conversation on the topic of Medical Generalism, Now! All the speakers then reviewed and revised the narrative to bring you the reported conversation that follows.

DOI: 10.1201/9781003297222-7

It is an incomplete conversation. We intentionally only explored whole person care in so-called Western medicine healthcare settings – our own areas of expertise. Yet, at a time when global healthcare urgently needs to change, we should not ignore the potential opportunities created by cross-cultural conversations. There are just six experts in the field around this virtual table – meaning there are many more voices to be heard. This first conversation perhaps lays some of the foundations for those discussions still to come.

7.2 INTRODUCING THE SPEAKERS

Let me introduce you to the five people who joined me around the table.

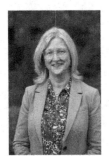
Prof Jane Gunn
Australia

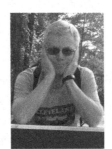
Prof Kurt Stange
USA

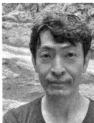
Dr Koki Kato
Japan

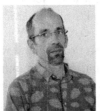
Dr Stefan Hjorleifsson
Norway

Prof Chris van Weel
The Netherlands

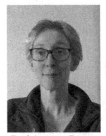
Prof Joanne Reeve
UK

Now, let the conversation begin!

7.3 GETTING STARTED: SETTING THE SCENE

Joanne: Thank you all for joining this conversation to explore the knowledge work of advanced generalist practice. Having spent 20 years studying this topic, there are perhaps two things that stand out for me. First, the importance of knowledge work, which we'll come to shortly. But secondly, the impact of the context in which that work happens. So that's where I'd like to start – by understanding the healthcare setting in which generalist care happens in your country.

In the UK, general practice is free to access for all patients registered with that practice. Practices are staffed by multidisciplinary teams which include GPs, practice nurses, advanced clinical practitioners, physician associates, pharmacists and others, with administrative support. In most cases, patients can only access specialist care if they are referred by their GP. General practices are contracted by the NHS to provide primary care services – a baseline service to everyone for a per capita fee, with incentivised additional items of service (e.g., screening, chronic disease management) as determined by the national contract. How does that compare with where you are all working?

Koki: In Japan, healthcare costs are covered by public insurance and a per-service co-payment of between 10% and 30% depending on income, while medical services are provided by private institutions. Patients can freely access physicians in any specialities, not just general practice or primary care. Primary care teams usually consist of physicians, nurses and clerks. GP training in Japan is 3 or 4 years. We work in small teams and generally we do not have nurse practitioners. Physicians are free to open their own clinic. Primary care services may be provided by physicians with other specialty training. Patients pay a fee to see their chosen clinician. For my clinic to be viable, I need to see about forty patients in a day.

Kurt: In the US, there is no guarantee of healthcare, although emergency departments have to take people in. It's an insurance-based healthcare system. People who are working have insurance through their employers. The government is still the biggest provider of insurance through Medicare, which covers almost everybody who is 65 years and over, and people with disabilities. Medicaid, which is administered at the state level, is for poor people. And then we still have probably 10% of our people uninsured.

There are very diverse approaches to primary care. It's generally thought to be provided by family physicians, and also general internists, general paediatricians, nurse practitioners and physician assistants. Training for family physicians takes 3 years, with some people trying to increase this to 4 years. Around half of our primary care physicians are now employed by large vertical care systems with a great loss of autonomy for individual clinicians. But with larger practices come multidisciplinary teams including behavioural and mental healthcare. But there's a great shortage of primary care. One of the tenants of primary care is accessibility. It's very difficult to get in and that really makes it difficult for us to do a lot of what we're supposed to do. One interesting innovation is 'Direct Primary Care'. People pay a monthly subscription fee and for that get all their primary care. It's not common, but it's an innovative model that's growing. It ranges from single-handed practices that provide all for a fee to very large multispecialty practices.

Joanne: There's already so much here that is clearly going to shape the way we work with patients. What's it like in Australia, Jane?

Jane: At the heart of it is a fee-for-service system. Currently, we are at a very point of crisis in Australian healthcare workforce needs. General practice works as a recognised specialty – general practice training is a postgraduate qualification and GPs are expected to have that. We do have an accreditation process for practices as well, but that is not compulsory. There's no patient registration. It is a blended system for payments. GPs are in private businesses, although there are some exceptions. But the basic way it is supported is through a mix of fee-for-service and what we call blended payments, which are a whole host of other ways of paying either for individual services or for practice-based sort of incentive payments. It is a very complex system. It's not population based.

Since the 1990s, there's been a lot of work to implement a quality improvement process within general practice. GPs undergo a continuing professional development process where they update every 3 years. They're required to do certain stuff to keep up to date and some of that does focus on quality improvement processes within the practice. There are a lot of guidelines, there's the College of GPs' guideline document called the *Red Book*. They're held up as best practice and some are incentivised, if you like, through payment mechanisms.

Joanne: Finance, and the business side of general practice delivery, is a really strong thread here. Chris and Stefan, what's it like where you are?

Chris: The Netherlands is broadly similar to the UK. We also have a practice-based list of patients and the practice will deliver healthcare when needed and refer to specialist care in the minority of cases that that is needed. We have an entirely privately insured health system. Everyone is obliged to take health insurance and every health insurance scheme has to have to work through primary care as the point of entry. So family physicians have a contract with the insurer for every patient on their list. There's probably less of a truly multidisciplinary team in every practice. There is a main emphasis on receptionists and the task of the receptionist, particularly in terms of continuity of care, is not adequately recognised. Nursing is available, but the links between family doctors and nursing facilities is very varied. Family physicians work in groups to cover 24-hour service, nights, weekends, and so on.

Stefan: In Norway, healthcare is tax funded so there is no insurance involved. GPs get a capitation and fee for service payment. The patient also pays a small sum each time they come, except children up to the age of 18. But there is a cap on how much someone has to pay in a year – after that, you don't pay anything. General practice is not multidisciplinary – mainly GPs and secretaries. I agree with Chris, secretaries are crucial. Norway has nursing, pharmacy and physiotherapists but they are not integrated. The key distinction between the UK and Norway is that you are listed with a designated GP – so we have personal continuity, not just practice continuity. We have just published some wonderful research on the benefits of continuity of care.

Joanne: So it's clear that there are lots we have in common – the commitment to whole person care, delivered where we can through the core principles of primary care (continuous, comprehensive, coordinated, accessible, person-centred care). But with big differences in the practical delivery of primary care in context – how we work with other medical disciplines, other healthcare specialties, healthcare funders and policy makers and our communities. There are lots of implications for knowledge work in practice from all that, so let's look a bit closer.

Considering knowledge work

Joanne: My book outlines the distinct knowledge work of advanced generalist practice. I have described it as the tailored, whole person exploration, explanation and evaluation of illness. It is this work which allows the generalist physician to safely and effectively work beyond disease or guideline boundaries to manage undifferentiated and complex care. I have also argued that this work is not adequately recognised, valued, understood or supported in modern UK healthcare; and that this needs to change. So I start by asking, do you recognise the ideas presented in this book? Are they relevant to general practice and primary care in your context?

Kurt: Yes, I recognise it. And where it's helpful, I think is that people often think the general practice is simple. They look at a list of the most common diseases that we have – sore throats, cold – okay, that's easy. Hypertension, diabetes, high cholesterol – okay, we have protocols for that – that's easy. And what they don't realise is that people come in with three or four of those things in one go, and new complaints, and mental health problems. Eighteen percent of patient visits have a family problem brought up. I think it is not understood that we scan all these things that are going on, to say what's the most important at this moment. And then across these different things, how do you integrate care, how do you choose maybe one treatment that works for two chronic diseases and helps their acute complaint today? So I think emphasising the knowledge work is about helping people understand the complexity of what we do, and the importance of it for the individuals and for the system. That prioritising function doesn't happen in a whole person way anywhere else in our healthcare system.

Yet, we devalue knowledge work in how we pay. If you're in a procedural oriented specialty, you make three or four times as much money. When I perform a procedure with someone – like freeze some skin tags – I get paid more than for caring for three chronic diseases and in two acute complaints in one visit.

Joanne: Do we perhaps also place greater value on the practical stuff in the way we ourselves think as a discipline of family medicine and general practice too? We don't see knowledge work as part of that practical work? We place great value on things like consultation skills (communication skills, relationship-based care). We have done lots of work to describe what those skills are, and dedicate much energy to teaching them to new clinicians. Yet, the underlying intellectual work that we do is often, in my experience, described simply as 'gut instinct' or 'tacit knowledge'. So we know we are doing it, but we don't perhaps value it enough to afford it the same attention as we pay to those other aspects of our practice? I have often had conversations with colleagues who have described these conversations as 'too academic' – which means it's not seen as part of the daily work of 'jobbing GPs'.

Kurt: Yes, I think very much so. When I went into the field, it was very much about the practical orientation – being pragmatic and practical. Research was something that was not relevant – and as a discipline, we've had a hard time developing a research base because of that idea. I think it's less with the newer generation, but I think is definitely part of the culture and the self-identity of our discipline.

Joanne: Interesting, thank you, Kurt. So how does a 'knowledge work' conversation sound in Japan, Koki?

Koki: I think it is useful to focus specifically on the knowledge work of generalist practice because it can help make the contrast between usual generalist and usual specialist practice. So when we provide general practice, the government and others can see what we are doing is usual practice, and also different from a specialist approach. So I like this idea – knowledge work is a very important viewpoint.

Joanne: And for you, Jane? You have led thinking on generalist practice, delivery and teaching for many years. How does a knowledge work perspective sound to you?

Jane: Yes, I recognise the idea too. I also think it is difficult to nail down, which I suppose is why it's a missing piece, as you say. It's easy to diminish the importance of it because we don't see it. That invisibility of what GPs do is part of our challenge – most of our conversations happen in private.

Joanne: So the system needs to trust the practitioner in that 'invisible space' to have the expertise to be able to make sense of a problem, put an action in place, follow it up and evaluate it, and amend if we need to? The work John Gabbay described as creating knowledge-in-practice-in-context, because externally created guidelines or pathways of care won't be enough to deal with the complexity of problems we see. How do we recognise, evaluate and reward that work? We spoke earlier about rewarding (paying) general practice for specific tasks, items of service. But how do we recognise and reward work that is invisible? But do you think, in principle, Australian health-care systems recognise this complex knowledge work as a legitimate part of healthcare?

Jane: I think at one level, it would be recognised as a legitimate role that general practice could play. I don't know if it would be written down, but I would agree that was an ideal that we were wanting from our GPs. Where it gets more complicated is not so much at the level of government policy documents, but in the lived experience of the healthcare system – what's actually happening in real life. It seems to me that there's been a reduction in trust in the medical profession – not so much from patients but from our governing and oversight bodies. But I also think the voice of the generalist is not on the same level of the voice of the specialists.

Joanne: Lord Moran's ladder still holds true then? In the UK in the 1960s, the Chair of the NHS Awards Committee, Lord Moran, described GPs as 'doctors who had fallen off the specialist ladder' (Reeve et al., 2013). But that aside, is there a way we can deal with that – challenge and change those perceptions?

Jane: Yes, I think so. In my work here in Australia to describe the role of the generalist in modern and future primary care systems, we described the similarities between the roles of generalist physician and a Chief Executive Officer (CEO). The hallmark of a good CEO is that they're a generalist – that they can see multiple perspectives and find effective ways to deal with complex situations. But you don't hear people saying, well, we're not going to listen to the CEO. So if you look at what makes an effective CEO – teamwork, learning new things, creativity, strong communication skills, scholarship – those are the functions of an effective GP generalist. There's medical knowledge that that the generalist has to manage, and of course, we see health very broadly. So we're often thinking about things that go into the social and relational domain and all of that. But there's a lot of other knowledge – management of care over time, the complex person in the context of their community, the weighing up of making decisions. That work is a balancing act and it's a different philosophy too.

Joanne: That brings another concept from the management and business theory world into these discussions, Jane, thank you. Much of the study of the concept of knowledge work comes from outside of healthcare too. It's great to be recognising that some of the creative ideas that may help us with current challenges lie in many spaces. I'd be interested to hear more about the experiences in Europe too. Stefan?

Stefan: So I totally recognise this idea of generalist expertise as the ability to work beyond guidelines and evidence in order to tailor healthcare to the individual in front of them. From my own professional perspective. And this is what I try to teach the undergraduates, the GP trainees and so on. But is it recognised as a central element of the Norwegian healthcare system and so pivotal to general practice? No. I wouldn't say so. We are recognised as gatekeepers. There's the personal continuity of care. But the generalist competence to manage beyond guidelines – no, I don't think that's well recognised here, no.

Chris: So I don't think it is recognised here in the Netherlands either. I think that it's going against all the bureaucratic ideas that you even dare to act against guidelines. GPs are the experts in acting beyond or outside guidelines? It's not recognised. It's probably part of what people do. It is probably part of what patients intuitively like.

Stefan: Yes, yes.

Chris: But it's not recognised because continuity is a word a bit like love. Everyone knows what it means, but no one is able to define it.

Joanne: So when you talk about continuity, you are referring to the whole-person-in-context perspective of expert generalist practice?

Chris: Yes. We can always define specialist knowledge, and as a consequence, the specialist knowledge takes precedence over the integrated approach to individuals. But I would say it is conceptually impossible not to be a generalist because I've never seen an individual with one single problem that can be solved by one single specialist. Individuals are complex. Health is part of that complexity. And that's one of the great things that this book is daring to enter into. We have to articulate the continuity of advanced generalist care beyond the fact that it is just seeing the same individual over and over again.

At this moment in my career, I'm often involved in reviewing and advising when mistakes have been made. I see examples of Family Doctors who have seen the same patient time and again. And continues to make the same mistake, time and again. So we have to understand the intellectual challenge that underpins continuity of whole person care because it is at the core of any part of medicine and it is impossible to be in primary care without.

Stefan: Yes, I think I can add from the Norwegian perspective there is a rising general practice workforce crisis. Our hospital managers recognise this and are looking to help. Politicians recognise that we need strong primary care and therefore continuity and personnel to be able to uphold the gatekeeping function. But that does not include recognition of the sophisticated generalist. We teach it, but that does not mean that it is recognised.

Joanne: So you are both flagging the importance of continuity. It's one of the five key elements of strong primary care, which Kringos's work shows delivers efficient, effective and equitable healthcare. But you also recognise that we need to be clearer about what we mean by continuity – what it is, why it matters. In the UK, we have traditionally put a lot of emphasis on relational continuity but I think you are flagging up something more?

Chris: It is an intellectual challenge to understand what it is we do. I don't think you can have good continuity of care if there is no relation, but the relation in itself is not continuity of care. Continuity of care is looking in a continuous way at the values for individuals, their understanding, demands, desires, preferences, and looking at various health problems at different moments in time through the lens of the whole person. I don't think we have a fundamental issue with guidelines. As a tool, they can be helpful. But a guideline is not solving this. The solutions we create are reflections of the values of the patient and the values of the doctor. Some of the things people may want, I would not be very happy to provide. So it is this interaction.

Joanne: What I describe in Chapter 2 is the co-creation of an Explanation of a problem. Drawing on multiple sources of information – from the patient, the practitioner and the guidelines – but ultimately to create something new, a tailored explanation in context – new knowledge-in-context.

Stefan: This resonates with our concerns in Norway. We have an issue with how national guidelines are produced – by expert groups, but working in silos and dominated by specialists. The generalist expertise not heard as relevant. We've been producing evidence here describing the over treatment that results from following guidelines, but it's not yet changing the way guidelines are made.

Joanne: Already this conversation is throwing up some really important issues for future, and current, healthcare – especially primary healthcare. If we want person-centred primary care, we need generalist practice. But we will need to get better at describing it so *other people* can understand it – so the generalist perspective can be an equal partner at the table when we're deciding what healthcare we need and deliver in our societies. We're trying to share it with our trainees – with new generalist physicians coming through, but we're still not getting the message across to the key policy decision makers. Perhaps this also reflects that we struggle with finding a common language for this work within the community of generalist practitioners. None of you rejects the term *knowledge work*, and its description makes sense to you – resonates with your own understanding of generalist practice. But it perhaps isn't the wording that would usually come to mind. Chris uses 'continuity of care' to describe work that includes ideas I have been discussing in this book as 'knowledge work'. Maybe we don't need a new term, but instead need to review and revise existing language? Yet, I started this book highlighting the problems we have with much of our terminology for our everyday work – for example, general practice, general practitioner and generalist practice. Maybe it is time for some new language after all.

Interestingly though, it seems that our patients understand this form of care and indeed want this form of care. Have we done enough to mobilise this powerful voice for generalist care?

So we have some work to do on finding a shared language and narrative on generalist care. But our discussion so far has also flagged up wider issues – in the way we plan and run our healthcare systems. So let's have a closer look at some of those. My research consistently highlights four barriers to generalist practice in the UK: perceived lack of permission for this work, its prioritisation, professional skills and confidence, and supportive performance management. Do any of those exist in your own practice?

Koki: In Japan, we do not have a permission barrier, and we don't have any performance measure which affects your decisions. We are allowed to practice literately freely, and there is room for tailored care. However, we need to see many patients to maintain our practice income at a viable level. We usually have to see around 40 patients a day to maintain our clinic. So a specialist may see many patients but needs a fairly limited time with each. But our patients who need generalist practice have multimorbidity. It takes time. From this view, the medical internist is a very hard worker in Japan. The complex work of generalist practice is not prioritised in our healthcare system. Patients with few illnesses who can be seen in a short time will work best from a profit point of view. However, this system is entirely inappropriate for an aging society with many patients suffering from multimorbidity.

Joanne: So the pressure to deliver quick care in order to make enough money to pay your staff and yourself effectively becomes a hidden performance management tool? It effectively defines what best care is, and requires you to deliver it in order for your practice to be viable? It limits, or even prevents, generalist care?

Kurt: Yes, I recognise everything Koki says and the barriers you describe. If you work for a big system, the safe thing to do is follow the guidelines for the diseases, crank people through, and try to make people happy. That's what you're evaluated on – your productivity: How many people do you see in a day, how many procedures did you do and did you do well on patient satisfaction? But every day, you see people that didn't fit any of the guidelines, and you have to go out of your way and go against some of the protocols. Sometimes, you take more time with them. I was trained to do that. Now, I think clinicians are more trained around protocols – and so they don't feel trained to deliver generalist care when it's needed.

Jane: In Australia, I think those barriers exist here as well. Performance appraisal is perhaps less of an issue here compared with the UK. But again, the emphasis is on productivity and billing. There's a big impetus for you to be in physical contact with a patient because you can't bill them too much otherwise. Whereas good generalist work happens outside the consultation. And so that's a huge gap here.

Stefan: In Norway, our fee-for-service includes payment for things like interdisciplinary meetings, but there there's no extra fee for managing multimorbidity. There is a fee for reviewing polyphar-macy, but nothing for managing multimorbidity in itself.

Joanne: There's a real theme here about productivity and moving people through the healthcare system. We have that issue too. In England, we are delivering around 33 million consultations with general prac-tice every month. We have a population of around 56 million people. Which means that more than half the population are visiting their general practice every month. The sheer volume of work is driving a very transactional model of healthcare delivery.

Chris: You need to have a GP who uses their mind – who is thinking, who is reflecting. How do we pay for the need to reflect?

Koki: Yes, this is a very important topic. We need the Wise Policy that you describe in your chapter, Joanne, to value and facilitate gen-eralist practice appropriately. We will need a significant shift in healthcare policy, including the payment system.

Joanne: So it sounds like the real barrier to generalist practice in action is the healthcare system – the context in which people are working. With both visible and hidden drivers pushing health professionals to behave in a particular way. Yet, you've all also described health pro-fessionals working 'under the radar' – delivering advanced generalist care despite of the system, rather than because of it? So where does this professional drive come from? Where do clinicians develop this sense of purpose, and the skills to do it? Is it part of your profes-sional training?

Koki: The knowledge work of general practice – yes, I think that is a part of professional postgraduate training in Japan. Family medi-cine training in my country includes some elements of the knowl-edge work. For example, the patient-centred clinical method by Stewart and others is widely known with GP trainers and trainees in Japan. So they usually have some knowledge about the impact of illness experience and context on how patients present. These are the fundamental elements in the knowledge work of generalist practice.

Joanne: That's great to hear. I think we touch on it too, but a far greater emphasis is placed on learning the guidelines. In conversations I have had with them, our GP trainers want to be able to explore the full range of professional practice. But first and foremost, they have to get their trainees through the exam system that allows them to qualify as a GP and then work. And the exam system is very geared towards: Do you know the guideline? Do you follow the guideline? So when and how do we learn the advanced skills to work safely and effectively beyond those guidelines?

Kurt: When I trained, it was very much focused on the pragmatics of delivering whole person care. But now I think that's changed. There's a lot more focus on evidence-based medicine, following protocols, and therefore on disease-focused care.

Stefan: In Norway, we don't have the problem that you are describing, Joanne. There are no exams that force the trainers to focus on specific ways of working that might align poorly with what the patient presents with. The main place where we discuss generalist skills with the trainees is in our trainee groups. So I'm a trainer and I meet once a month for a full day with eight or ten trainees. I do this every month for 2 years. And you can do quite sophisticated stuff in that time. They bring their everyday struggles from their clinical work and we agree on a paper to read and we apply that to the problems they are struggling with. We have a long discussion asking how does a good GP deal with this? What can we use the guideline for and what is the limits of the guideline?

Joanne: That sounds very similar to the CATALYST programme we run for newly qualified GPs, Stefan. You are helping them develop these skills before they enter general practice. Food for thought here, I think. Jane, you are Dean of the medical school at Melbourne. Do you think that these discussions, debates and ideas are discussed with undergraduate students with postgraduate students?

Jane: Not enough. There's a lot of focus on giving general practice more prominence. Because only 14% of our graduates go into general practice. In many areas of Australia, we're relying on international medical graduates to staff our clinics. Students get so inspired by the people that they see and work with in all of the areas that they are exposed to. But the generalist option is so disadvantaged for a whole lot of reasons. Students are not inspired by what they see of the generalist function. A journalist once asked me about fast tracking people to get to GP and giving them a really short, sharp training program to be a GP. And I thought therein lies a fundamental part of the problem – the assumption that the GP job is somehow easier and so can be learned in a short time.

Chris: I try to show students the complexity of generalist practice. What I did was to take a common health problem and with a clear guideline and then focus on three different patients with that same problem. For example, a sore throat. One person comes to you because they have severe health anxiety. Here, we must treat their anxiety, not (just) their sore throat. The second is going on a skiing holiday and worried about being ill whilst away. The third is different again. To show we have three different patients with, apparently, the same problem, and we do three completely different things. Well, that's where the generalist thinking starts because you focus on the context of the individual. For the doctor, or indeed the teacher working with a student, this way of thinking potentially puts them in a vulnerable position. Because they are analysing something of which s/he doesn't have a ready at hand answer all the time. I think that's what people find threatening. And I think that's what we have to overcome.

Joanne: Creating that knowledge-in-context-in practice that John Gabbay talks about. Its difficult work isn't it? But not recognised and valued.

Kurt: Yes, and when you combine the loss of professional autonomy that comes with top-down quality measures, with the productivity pressures to get as many people through as you can in a day, you can see why we face a big problem of burnout. To do whole person care with people, where you have to take a little extra time, it makes you look bad on your productivity measures and you can only do so much of that.

Joanne: The professional becomes just a cog in the wheel?

Kurt: Healthcare has become much more transactional, much less personal. The idea that it's a relationship is really gone and when you're being efficient – you can be efficient about transactions. But it's hard to be efficient about the relationship aspects or the personalising aspects of it. There's an arrogance from the top – we think we know what needs to be done and we just try to crank people through, do it as efficiently as we can and that's fine.

Joanne: And Koki, are you seeing or feeling those de-professionalisation elements in Japan? How does it feel for you?

Koki: Current GP trainers and trainees in Japan choose careers with a strong ambition to provide holistic healthcare, even though the recognition and field of GPs is underdeveloped as yet. Trained GPs can provide this care, even if they work under pressure to make a profit. But many primary care physicians working in Japan have not had primary care training at the undergraduate or postgraduate level. So our challenge is that we need to catch up.

Stefan: We don't have any specific support for mid-career GPs either. In Norway, you need to re-certify every 5 years and to do that you need to be part of a peer group that meets I think a minimum of four times a year. But I am not sure these provide the support of support we're talking about here. I've been discussing this with colleagues in academic general practice and thinking about the complexity and the weight of the decisions that need to be made every day. So you need to resist falling into a sort of single cause, single effect, single guideline and a linear causality way of thinking. But in order to resist that, you need to be part of an ongoing professional discussion. A fellowship sounds great.

Chris: In the Netherlands, every 5 years, your practice has to be reassessed. A couple of years ago, the Dutch College tried to change that to a complete practice audit, which was resisted initially. But when the practices started, their views changed. The new system brought them recognition from the college for all aspects of the way they ran their practice – an extensive audit of the practice running. I think that that is one way of getting out of the mode of we are siloed providers of predefined health problems with a predefined solution into looking at how do we organise and cope with the complexity of the work we do.

Joanne: Is there something there about professional leadership. Recognising we are not just technicians or deliver what someone else tells us, but a professional discipline in our own right who lead, as well as deliver, a distinct model of whole person care? Being publicly recognised for the complexity of the work we do?

Stefan: And by patients and the community too. In Norway, we are discussing a new collaborative project with the College. A national project to educate patients about how to use your general practice in a good way. So you don't go to your GP and say I need an MRI and a referral, or my mother said I need these pills. Instead, go to the GP and tell her about your worries, your symptoms and trust that the best thing you can get from your GP is her brain power. Her undivided attention is the best thing you can get. We talk about it as health literacy – to explain prudent use of general practice. Because nobody has ever explained this to people in Norway. At least for a few decades. And we are trying to turn that around. And it strikes me that we are explaining that you don't use general practice as a place where you order something. Instead, you use your GP's generalist skills.

Joanne: That's a really important conversation, Stefan – how we have this conversation with our patients, our communities. Help them to understand the value of a 'thoughtful' (and wise) GP.

Chris: Yes, and we need to broaden this too because generalist practice is also an important part of the intellectual performance of specialists and subspecialists. We tend to look at it as a job description – as a distinction between, say, GPs and hospital doctors. Where actually the real value of a specialist's work is related to the extent in which they are able to put that into a generalist approach with continuity and with consistency over time.

Joanne: I agree completely, Chris. I talk in Chapter 2 about generalist skills not being unique to a GP or defining a professional role. For a GP, they are part of a skill set. But I quote Stefan in his description of the GP role being defined by the ability to oscillate between a generalist whole person thinking and a specialist disease-focused thinking. If you're in practice and a person comes in with crushing chest pain, you need to use your specialist skills instantly. If they come in and cry, you may start with a generalist approach. That's what I teach to all our students.

Kurt: I like that you have a statement that says the goal of whole person medicine is enhancing health as a resource people need for daily living. I like that practical focus. But daily living could sound just mundane – just how you get through the day. And I think it's much more than that. We can help them to transcend their suffering, help them through some key life transitions. So there's something about championing and supporting that role too.

Koki: And that needs supervisors – trainers and mentors for qualified doctors – who are adequately trained to support and encourage this reflection. In Japan, many GP trainers know about Stewart's person-centred clinical method. However, from my perspective, a good number of supervisors only have experience in hospital-based medicine. I feel they cannot appropriately provide person-centred decision making because they may not adequately know or explore a patient's context. We need supervisors adequately trained to encourage reflection.

Joanne: Thank you both. I think you're highlighting that we need to adequately support doctors – trainees, yes, but also at all career stages – in this complex reflection that is core to whole person medicine. We can't just assume people know how to do it, or that they can and will be able to do it in their daily working lives. We need to build support for this work into the way we design primary care. That is the idea behind the Wise Hub I talk about in Chapter 6.

Jane: I think it's really important what you're doing here. And I also think it's urgent. We need to do more – put it to the forefront as a medical profession. One of the things I have sort of been lobbying for is excellent *clinical* leadership programs for GPs – raising the profile of GPs as healthcare leaders, not just people who deliver. And we need a sense of urgency for change.

Joanne: What a great point to bring this conversation to at least a temporary close, Jane. Thank you to you all for offering such a rich and fascinating glimpse into primary care and general practice in your contexts. And whilst there are certainly differences – for example in how we fund care, how we train practitioners – there is far more that is shared.

Perhaps most loudly, I am hearing the shared need to recognise, value and champion the complexity of the work of whole person, advanced generalist medicine. Your descriptions highlight how this work too often remains hidden, in all of our settings around the world. It is this hidden work which also lies at the core of our shared professional identity. And the failure to understand and champion this work is contributing to our universal challenge in encouraging people to come into, and stay working, in general practice.

I am struck by the impact of the infrastructure challenges that we all face and all share. Even though our services are funded differently, there seems to be a common 'business model' driving the work we do. Each of you describe the drive to complete work on time and on budget as shaping the clinical care we offer. Of course, services need to run to budget and deliver a standard. Maybe it is the way we define the budgets and standard that we are challenging. Again, that comes back to describing and championing the value of an alternative approach.

And again, you have described the importance of the continuing work to develop and maintain a whole person understanding of illness, and how best to manage it. I am intrigued by Jane's description of how this likens our work to the CEO. Like the CEO, the generalist keeps an eye on the goal (in our case, health for living). And has the knowledge, skills and expertise to continually navigate through a potentially changing landscape towards that goal. In other words, the essence of whole person knowledge work.

So thank you all for a conversation which underlines and expands ideas presented in this book, has introduced new ideas, and lies the foundations for many more conversations to come.

You can find more discussion of Lord Moran here:

Reeve J, Irving G, Freeman G. (2013). Dismantling Lord Moran's ladder: the primary care expert generalist. British Journal of General Practice, 63, pp. 34–35.

Index

Note: *Italicized* page numbers refer to figures in the text.

Printed in the United States
by Baker & Taylor Publisher Services